T0233451

Dr. Hales's *Healing the Healer* is both a personal journey and an analysis of the cost of being a healer. Her book is rich with story, rich with insight, rich with compassion. She is practical and pragmatic, and yet she also gives something rather metaphoric and poetic. One need not be a physician to be moved and enlarged by Hales's capacity to move through the valley of suffering to understanding, and to wisdom. How she works in a counselling capacity with physicians in distress is brilliant.

James Hollis, PhD, Jungian analyst and author of *Living Between Worlds: Finding Personal Resilience in Changing Times*

This book is a must read at a time when doctors and other medical professionals are dealing with an epidemic that demands we recognize the incredible toll it is taking on those who care for the sick, the dying, and their families. Suzanne Hales gives voice to those dedicated professionals who risk their own lives and suffer deep wounding as they work in the realm between life and death. Diving below the surface of the frozen heart, she opens the door of love and understanding, which allows the tears of healing to reach the wounds that are so often hidden from the world.

Janis M. Maxwell, *PhD, Training Analyst and Faculty of the C.G. Jung Institute in Zürich; Ex-President and Director of Training, Philadelphia Jung Institute; Ex-Director of Training, Inter-Regional Society of Jungian Analysts*

Dr. Hales brings to the writing of this excellent book the most advanced training in Jungian psychology, four decades of doing therapy with medical professionals, and her own fascinating story of healing and personal growth. Practitioners at all levels of the medical fields, as well as those who offer therapy to them, not only will be instructed by this book, but will also find it inspirational. The book is a powerful challenge to medical educators to prepare their students more adequately for the rigors of the unique demands of their profession.

James A. Kitchens, *PhD, Professor, University of North Texas*

Healing the Healer is the personal story of a therapist who for decades has treated the unspoken and often repressed suffering of physicians. By recounting their stories, Dr. Hales opens the reader to the dark traumas shielded from view behind a white coat, and the ways in which a Jungian therapist can open the suffering physician to paths of healing. As an emergency physician with forty years of experience, the stories recounted here echo the challenges I have witnessed repeatedly in my own life and in the lives of my fellow physicians. This is a book of healing that should be read by every therapist who works with physicians.

Lance S. Owens, *MD, Medical Doctor, University of Utah Medical Center; Attending Physician, Salt Lake City Veteran's Administration Medical Center; Editorial board member of Psychological Perspective, Journal of the C. G. Institute, Los Angeles, CA*

In her book, Suzanne Hales does not aim to change the culture of medicine, but rather to help the healer—the 21st-century doctor—find healing through integration as a whole physician, not just an outcomes-driven one. In this, she succeeds admirably. This is a necessary book that should be read by all practitioners and students in the healing professions.

Carl V. Boyer, *MD, Family Physician in New York, NY*

Healing the Healer provides profound insight regarding the dynamics of giving and receiving care in all realms of healthcare. Suzanne Hales offers her perspectives based on decades of clinical experience, and life experience, to ask important questions about the future of caring. It is a deep examination of the risks and the rewards of care and will benefit clinicians across disciplines who hope to provide healing to others and for themselves.

Betty Ferrell, *PhD, RN, FAAN, FPCN, Professor and Director of Nursing Research, City of Hope Medical Center, Los Angeles CA; Director, The End of Life Nursing Education Consortium (ELNEC) Project*

From its outset, it is clear this is a revolutionary book, one that is essential reading for anyone working in healthcare or interested in the inner world of physicians. The practical application of Jungian psychology, as related to physicians and other healers, was so instructive, and with brilliant, easily accessible writing, *Jungian Psychotherapy with Medical Professionals* shows how healing goes both ways, between the clinician and the patient. Hales's revolutionary insights offer hope and healing for the medical community and our healthcare system.

Elizabeth Ann Robinson, PhD, RN, CNS, author of *The Soul of the Nurse*
www.ElizabethAnnRobinson.com

This volume concerns the ups & downs of medicine, and the hopeful & hopeless nature of this rewarding & difficult work. There is nothing like welcoming a newborn into this world and assisting an ill and dying patient to accept the next phase of life's journey. While on the Admission Committees at UCSF, University of Rochester and Texas A&M University Schools of Medicine, I did my best to admit students of all backgrounds, such as art & music. Medicine has been slow to change, but the dramatic rise in the number of women in medicine has helped /helping immensely. When I graduated with an M.D. in 1970 there were 5% women, but now there are 50%.

This ten fold increase has helped medicine to become more feeling based and a more sensitive profession.

David H. Rosen, *M.D, Medical Doctor and Affiliate Professor in Psychiatry at Oregon Health and Science University in Portland, Oregon*

Jungian Psychotherapy with Medical Professionals

Jungian Psychotherapy with Medical Professionals guides therapists, clinicians, and healthcare workers through the transformative healing process of Jungian psychology, demonstrating how the new spirit of medicine will originate from the relationship between the healer and the healed.

Through extensive experience and scientific research gathered over the past four decades working closely with physicians, Suzanne Hales presents the telling of their stories that have been historically hushed or hidden away. Hales offers a lifeline for healthcare workers as she weaves together the stories of physicians and their patients with gripping honesty, presenting an intimate glimpse of what happens in the lives of healers and the healed. The book offers support to the healer in need of healing, provides hope for wholeness and restoration, and advocates for those who spend their lifetime advocating for others.

The book is of great interest to Jungian analysts, therapists, and trainees, and it is essential reading for anyone working in healthcare, including physicians and healers of all kinds in the landscape of modern medicine.

Suzanne Hales is a Swiss-trained Jungian analyst in private practice in McKinney, Texas. A licensed marriage and family therapist and professional counselor, she is also an international lecturer and storyteller. She is the President of the C.G. Jung Institute, Dallas Texas. She is the founder of Counseling and Consulting Associates of North Texas and the Crescent Moon Lodge and Retreat Center in the Kiamichi Wilderness in Oklahoma, where she leads workshops, trainings, and retreats.

Jungian Psychotherapy with Medical Professionals

Medical Professionals

Healing the Healer

Suzanne Hales

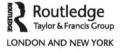
Routledge
Taylor & Francis Group

LONDON AND NEW YORK

Cover image: Cover art by Debra Worrell Hernandez

First published 2022
by Routledge
2 Park Square, Milton Park, Abingdon, Oxon OX14 4RN

and by Routledge
605 Third Avenue, New York, NY 10158

Routledge is an imprint of the Taylor & Francis Group, an informa business

© 2022 Suzanne Hales

The right of Suzanne Hales to be identified as author of this work has been asserted accordance with sections 77 and 78 of the Copyright, Designs and Patents Act 1988.

All rights reserved. No part of this book may be reprinted or reproduced or utilised in any form or by any electronic, mechanical, or other means, now known or hereafter invented, including photocopying and recording, or in any information storage or retrieval system, without permission in writing from the publishers.

Trademark notice: Product or corporate names may be trademarks or registered trademarks, and are used only for identification and explanation without intent to infringe.

British Library Cataloguing-in-Publication Data
A catalogue record for this book is available from the British Library

Library of Congress Cataloging-in-Publication Data
A catalog record has been requested for this book

ISBN: 978-0-367-70083-6 (hbk)
ISBN: 978-0-367-70084-3 (pbk)
ISBN: 978-1-003-14450-2 (ebk)

DOI: 10.4324/9781003144502

Typeset in Times New Roman
by MPS Limited, Dehradun

To Randall, thank you for your love for me, the many sacrifices you made, and your continual support of the work I do.

To my children and grandchildren—Kelli, Emilee, Stephen, Cole, Landrie, Randall, McKenzie, and Charlee Grace—thank you.

To Dr. Samuel Lifshitz and to Patrice Gilmore...

Dr. Lifshitz, you both inspired me and terrified me. You asked hard questions. Your kindness, curiosity, encouragement, and toughness were exemplified as you participated in this process with me. For all you have given me, my deepest thanks.

Patrice Gilmore, my late friend, your encouragement helped me hold on to these ideas until they could take written form. Thank you for your unwavering love and support.

Contents

Figures

Foreword

Medicine is an empirical science, which means that practical experience is more important than theoretical ideas. During the Enlightenment, the Renaissance idea that every science could in a rational way "enlighten" every problem flourished. It was a great achievement, when humans were able to weigh and measure, and this triumph over the arbitrary still lies in the background of any science.

However, the human mind is not only rational; it is also irrational, and the irrational holds many of our feelings and is the source of creativity. Only by putting away the narrow shields of rationality and irrationality can a whole immense new field of understanding be opened. Certainly science helps us to understand the world of existence, but experience is often beyond comprehension. I believe there is divine purpose. I don't like illnesses, but they are a fact with which I have to reckon. As I am a medical doctor, who is called to this profession, I am challenged by them. I think the current coronavirus pandemic shows us our basic task: is my task to keep the population healthy, as with every illness, or is my task to conquer the coronavirus, to fight it off so that it disappears? This is a central question for every physician. Am I so powerful as to win this battle with the disease, or am I to concede to the power of the illness and only help the patient to survive it?

These moral questions are not dealt with in the auditoriums of medical schools. My question, whether a disease can be meaningful, is rarely, if ever, asked. The task of the medical doctor is to heal, end of discussion! But what if the illness is stronger than the medical practitioner? In former times when practitioners could recognize the limits of their power, when they were defeated, they handed patients over to the nurses who would accompany them to death. These days much more is possible. Practitioners are more reluctant to surrender. With modern surgical techniques, anesthesia, and pharmaceuticals, so much can be achieved that was inconceivable before. But we must ask this question anew: where are the limits?

Suzanne Hales had to suffer the limits herself in order to understand this question. This makes her book unique. Not every practitioner has had to suffer an illness to understand what the patient is enduring. But because she has through this same hell, she can understand a patient's suffering.

She was called to be a medical practitioner; however, her father initially prevented her from pursuing this profession. Perhaps this caused her to suffer disease herself. Her unconscious called her to this profession. Since antiquity medicine has been a dangerous profession at the limits of Life and Death. To my mind, it requires a religious attitude in connection with the Divine to perform it properly. Dr. Hales experienced the abyss of the profession and she survived. The stories she tells here—her own and those of other medical practitioners—are not heard in medical schools.

My task in writing this foreword is to emphasize to the reader the value of Dr. Hales's unique perspective. She offers not only her outer experience, but also an original understanding from the inside of illness. In this way she encompasses the whole. The possibility of seeing the facts from both sides provides a more complete image, going much deeper into the essence of illness.

I hope that many medical practitioners will benefit from her experience in their daily work, gaining an understanding of their patients at a more fundamental level. This would be to the good of the patient, in particular, and of medicine, in general.

Alfred Ribi, MD

Acknowledgments

To those of you who have supported, encouraged, inspired me, and helped sustain me in writing this book, thank you.

To Dr. James Kitchens who introduced me to the work of Carl Jung, thank you.

I have a great sense of gratitude for those men and women called physicians, who have trusted me with their process—a debt that can never be repaid, only acknowledged. Thank you. Your willingness to let me witness your lives has opened my heart to a deeper level, and I am still not sure who heals whom. To those of you who have given me permission to share your stories, I am deeply appreciative. The names used in this book have all been changed to protect the privacy of the physicians.

Dr. Murray Fox, the "first physician" that I worked with to bring depth psychology to the world of medicine, although a completely foreign concept to the medical profession in the early 1980s, sparked the experience and research documented in this book. Thank you for trusting me with your colleagues and practice.

Dr. Elizabeth Coronado, Dr. Dennis Eisenberg, Dr. Daryl Greebon, Dr. Jules Monier, Dr. David Baghdassarian, Dr. Shuchi Desai, Dr. Quyen Dang, Dr. Benjamin Downie, Dr. Phil Bechtel, Dr. Michael Escamilla, Dr. Winston Marshall, Dr. DeAn Strobel, Dr. Michael Pfaff, Dr. Andrew Murphy, Dr. Ari Reddy, Dr. Robert Pollack, Dr. Scott Kemp, and Dr. May Mokbelpur, Dr. Bill Entzminger, Dr. Charu Chandrasekaran, Dr. Lance Owens, Dr. Carl Boyer, who listened, who asked questions, who read and reread and shared many words of wisdom and encouragement.

To my staff at CCA, Val Thompson, Jason Dehner, Rachel Dehner, and Kelli Smart.

To Alana Calhoun, Carol Smith, Brandi Sellers, and Daniel Porter, thank you for your help as this book was taking its first form.

To my publishing editor-in-chief Susannah Frearson, thank you for believing in this book and guiding me to its publication. LeeAnn Pickrell for your editing and project management, bringing structure and form, and to Angie Woods who went way beyond the call of duty in moving this material from thesis form to book form.

To my dear friends and colleagues, Richard Abernathy, Jennifer Embry, James Gossett, Cheryle Van Skoy, Renee Cobb, Cheryl Soignier, Donna Cozort, Tess Castleman, Daniel Renate, David Genty, Melissa Werner, Barbara Weskamp, Jean-Jacques Faber, Patti Carr, Stephanie Whisenhunt, Gene Baker, Chloe Schneider, Trenna Blalock, Clay Brantley, Silberia Garcia, Mark Kuban, Heather Biehunko, Michelle Bernard, Dave Eubanks, Linda Sprague, Joan Schroeder, George Petriccione, Rebecca and Chuck Culverson, and Shelly Glasner.

To the C. G. Jung Institute, Kusnacht, Switzerland, for my training and without which *Jungian Psychotherapy with Medical Professionals* would not have been "birthed."

To artist Debra Worrell Hernandez for creating a brilliant book cover and to Linda Phillips for your many art designs along the way.

To Dr. Janis Maxwell who was instrumental in honoring my unique perspective of this world. Your kindness and grace are like the softness of a cool gentle breeze that always invites me back to the springtime, thank you.

To Dr. Robert Hinshaw who introduced me to the beauty of the ancestors of the Jungian community, having traveled before me and inviting me to embrace the vastness of the work of Carl Jung and the meaning of the call of analyst, thank you.

To Dr. Alfred Ribi who has been a strong and mighty rock while having the waters of the lake at your feet. You created a safe temenos as you held my dreams and tears, while you guided me. The many conversations and endless questions we explored were an invitation to find my own authentic voice. You were strong enough to let me find my way, however long it took. I am especially thankful for the affirmation of my work as you often said, "This work is important work." You and Kelly were close and trusted guides along the way.

Credits

Epigraph in Prologue republished with permission of White Pine Press, from Antonio Machado, *There Is No Road*, translated by Dennis Maloney and Mary Berg, 2003.

Epigraph in Chapter One republished with permission of New York University Press, from Erich M. Remarque, *All Quiet on the Western Front*, translated by Brian Murdoch.

Epigraph in Chapter Two republished with permission of Routledge / Taylor & Francis Group, from "The Psychology of the Transference" (pp. 163–201), *The Practice of Psychotherapy*, by C.G. Jung, Vol. 16, of *The Collected Works of C. G. Jung*, 1965.

Epigraph in Chapter Four republished with permission of Princeton University Press, from *Psychology and Alchemy*, by C.G. Jung, Vol. 12, of *The Collected Works of C. G. Jung*, 1980. permission conveyed through Copyright Clearance Center, Inc.

Epigraph in Chapter Five republished with permission of Routledge / Taylor & Francis Group, from "Foreword to the Fourth Swiss Edition" (pp. xxiii–xvii), *Symbols of Transformation*, by C.G. Jung, Vol. 5, of *The Collected Works of C. G. Jung*, 1956.

Epigraph in Chapter Six from *The Red Book* by C.G. Jung, edited by Sonu Shamdasani, translated by Mark Kyburz, John Peck, and Sonu Shamdasani. Copyright © 2009 by the Foundation of the Works of C.G. Jung. Translation copyright © 2009 by Mark Kyburz, John Peck, and Sonu Shamdasani. Used by permission of W.W. Norton & Company. Inc.

Epigraph in Chapter Eight republished with permission of Spring Publications Adolph Guggenbühl-Craig, *Power in the Healing Professions*, 1971.

Epigraph in Chapter Nine republished with permission of Princeton University Press, from *Analytical Psychology: Notes of the Seminar Given in 1925*, by C.G. Jung, 1988, permission conveyed through Copyright Clearance Center, Inc.

Epigraph in Chapter Thirteen is from the book *Soulcraft*. Copyright © 2003 by Bill Plotkin. Reprinted with permission of New World Library, Novato, CA. www.newworldlibrary.com.

William Stafford, "The Way It is," from *Ask Me: 100 Essential poems*. Copyright © 1977, 2004 by William Stafford and the Estate of William Stafford. Reprinted with the permission of the Permissions Company, LLC, on behalf of Graywolf Press, Minneapolis, Minnesota, www.graywolfpress.com.

Excerpt from "Burnt Norton" from *Collected Poems 1909–1962* by T.S. Eliot. Copyright © 1952 by Houghton Mifflin Harcourt Publishing Company, renewed 1980 by Esme Valerie Eliot. Reprinted by permission of Houghton Mifflin Harcourt Publishing Company. All rights reserved.

Prologue

There is no path. The path must be forged as you walk.
Antonio Machado, *There Is No Road*

My personal story began 68 years ago. Three years ago, I had a dream that changed the trajectory of my life. The dream awakened me out of a deep sleep. In the liminal space just before sunrise, the time that connects the darkness to the light, the imaginal world of the dream, synchronicities, and divine guidance of the unconscious had a hand in weaving together the threads that formed the very fabric of my life that asked me to change, as I held onto the words of Carl Jung: "All true things must change and only that which changes remains true" (1963, p. 358, para. 503).

This research would take my unfinished business from childhood and, in a demanding and disruptive way, press me toward a task I would certainly want to run away from; however, I was more afraid not to run to it.

All change is difficult, both societal change and individual change. At the present time we are experiencing great disruption in all the major institutions. Institutions such as the educational, religious, and political as well as the institution of medicine, are in the middle of enormous flux. We are in the midst of a time of death and renewal. What makes change difficult is that, on the one hand, we find ourselves unwilling to release the old. And, on the other hand, we are afraid because we do not know what the new will bring. Also, change requires new ideas, new people, and a new spirit to emerge when the old structure is no longer in service to humanity. Blame can be placed on the government, insurance companies, medical schools, greed, or whatever evil we choose, or we can take a look at the old myths and see that whatever was great at one time must die for new life to come forth. We desperately need help in the creation of the new kingdom of medicine that is to come. It is my hope that this manuscript contributes to the coming of new life for the field of medicine and all its practitioners, including nurses, hospital aides, social workers, psychologists, medical researchers, and faculty members who are training these practitioners.

DOI: 10.4324/9781003144502-101

Among medical professionals, personal change is often necessary, but difficult because of their positions and status of practicing all types of medicine. There is an array of opposing tensions in the world of the physician. They are pulled between two worlds in many ways. Ego and soul, psyche and soma, doing and being, masculine and feminine, conscious and unconscious, the list goes on ad infinitum. I hear the stories of the torn curtain in the interior life that is lived in the external demands of the physician. Many of them are torn apart, unable to grow or move beyond their wounds and fragmentation. This book embarks on the task of entering these tensions and of exploring the pain rather than running from it, hiding from it, or splitting it off. We are called to unify this split, to know and experience wholeness... The poet Kahlil Gibran (1923) wrote, "Your joy is your sorrow unmasked. The self-same well from which your laughter rises was often times filled with your tears... the deeper the sorrow carves into your being the more joy you can contain." Our interior investigations and integrations are the soul-making task of our lives. It is this process of soul making that gives meaning to the suffering of being human.

I am not sure what really heals; that remains a mystery. I do know through experience that reflection and imagination are some of the things that set healing in motion. In that process there is in all of us a constant longing for contact with the numinous, however, you want to describe it... nature, energy, higher power, God, light, force, presence... we are wired that way. The seeking of connection is in our hard drive. These stories (mine and theirs) reveal a hunger, to be seen, to be heard, to be known, a connection between the known and the unknown with something larger than ourselves. It is a need with which we are born; it is our humanity. It is important to note that the names of all my patients throughout the book have been changed for their protection and privacy.

This work can apply not only to physicians but to anyone who holds presence for others in a healing capacity. Whether it be physicians, teachers, nurses, and other health professionals—anyone who holds the life of another in their hands. Carl Jung suggests we are tasked with helping others find their way against the backdrop of a system that fights desperately to keep that system in place, no matter how destructive that process may be. Perhaps better said,

> In the last analysis, every life is the realization of a whole, that is, of a self, for which reason this realization can also be called individuation. All life is bound to individual carriers who realize it, and it is simply inconceivable without them. But every carrier is charged with an individual destiny and destination, and the realization of this alone makes sense of life... if we respond to this it becomes our daemon, if not, the unlived life becomes the demon of our existence. (Jung 1968, p. 222, para. 330)

I do not think we are going to change the culture of medicine. My hope is we can find a different way of dealing with medicine and its impact on the lives it touches, both the physician and the patient. While we cannot, in ourselves, force the medical institution to change, I am convinced on the basis of 36 years of treating physicians and other medical personnel that we can help the healer find healing.

COVID-19: The pandemic

This book was completed in early February 2020. This was before the effects of COVID-19 were apparent, and before an unprecedented wave of trauma swept across all areas of our society, impacting every aspect of our lives. What struck the medical world at this time was unfathomable. Many articles and news stories have appeared even in the popular press with titles like "Emergency Physicians: Pandemic Compounds Stress of Difficult Job" (Hogberg, 2020, p. 43). What had been taboo to speak about was now at the forefront.

Hogberg quotes Dr. Alicia Terry of George Washington University School of Medicine and Health Sciences, "At moments it has been surreal and un-believable. It has been quite taxing physically as well as emotionally." Further, he quotes Dr. Mohamed Hagahmed, physician and faculty member at the University of Texas at San Antonio, "This pandemic has shown how vulnerable we are to emotional and mental stress." He closes the article with Dr. Hagahmed's statement, "I have not sought any professional help, but I need to."

People experience trauma when unwanted change forces its way into a person's life and they are forced into a situation over which they have no control. These experiences illicit feelings of helplessness for both participants and observers. COVID-19 has been traumatic for physicians as they have experienced a total sense of frustration and helplessness that so many pa-tients could not be saved. Through this pandemic, physicians are finding themselves in an inner conflict, regarding their morals and values, even their oath as they are being forced to make choices during this time that are often inhumane. This can, and sometimes does, lead to moral injury. Some of the identifiable symptoms of trauma include detachment, demoralization, in-ability to self-forgive, as they continue to experience the replay of the sounds, the replay of the relentless images and thoughts turned against themselves. The feelings of guilt, shame, fear, anger, and silent rage are often turned into self-punishing behaviors. The physical, mental, and emotional hours of this type of stress are daunting.

This pandemic has caused a breakdown in our daily structure and sense of security. Some have experienced the loss of jobs, social contacts, and even financial despair, illness, and death for both medical personnel, their families, and their patients. This pandemic has also brought attention and shed light on the fact that we are all vulnerable by our very nature of being human. Vulnerability, a word that was once associated by many as weakness, is now seen more accurately. Vulnerability simply means the possibility of being hurt. It has nothing to do with weakness; it is a mere fact of our shared humanity. This book is about that humanness.

We cannot heal ourselves by staying silent. Being able to feel safe with another person is probably the single most important aspect of mental health. It is a fundamental need, to be seen and to be heard. When this happens, safe connections are created, which are fundamental to meaningful and satisfying lives. This book is about relatedness, that of being truly heard and seen by the people around us. It is an inherent need in all of us, knowing and feeling that we are held in someone else's mind and heart. This experience opens the path for resilience-when we can be understood by and feel loved and attuned by the other. Physicians are in need of this healing now more than ever.

Jung concluded that within each of us is a deep resilience that he referenced as a divine spark that serves as a source of internal guidance. This is independent of our ego consciousness. We are all born with this capacity but we often forget until a crisis occurs which we can no longer control. My hope is that the crisis brought on by this pandemic may illuminate the needs of physicians and healthcare workers everywhere in our world, as we each call upon the divine spark within.

Suzanne Hales LPC LMFT Jungian Analyst EdD, Crescent Moon Retreat Center, Kiamichi Wilderness, Southeastern Oklahoma, October 1, 2020

References

Gibran, K. (1923). *The prophet*. New York, NY: Alfred A. Knopf.

Hogberg, D. (2020, August 18). Emergency physicians: pandemic compounds stress of difficult job. *Washington Examiner*, p. 43.

Jung, C.G. (1963). *The collected works of C. G. Jung: Vol. 14. Mysterium coniunctionis*. R.F.C. Hull (Trans.). H. Read, M. Fordham, G. Adler, & W. McGuire (Eds.). Princeton, NJ: Princeton University Press.

Jung, C.G. (1968). *The collected works of C. G. Jung, Vol. 12. Psychology and alchemy*. R.F.C. Hull (Trans.). H. Read, M. Fordham, G. Adler, & W. McGuire (Eds.). Princeton, NJ: Princeton University Press.

Machado, A. (2003). *There is no road: Proverbs by Antonio Machado*. D. Malony and M. Berg (Trans.). Buffalo, NY: White Pines Press.

Chapter 1

We are alone

It is a strange thing that all the memories have these two qualities. They are always full of quietness, that is the most striking thing about them; and even when things weren't like that in reality, they still seem to have that quality. They are soundless apparitions, which speak to me by looks and gestures, wordless and silent—and their silence is precisely what disturbs me.
Erich Maria Remarque, *All Quiet on the Western Front*

The bleeding began an hour after the baby was born.

Dr. Rhea's patient went to the hospital for induction of labor at 40 weeks. The induction went well, but after her patient had been completely dilated and pushing for three hours, Dr. Rhea made a decision with her patient for a C-section. Due to a lack of adequate staffing and an OB emergency, the patient had to wait another three hours to get into the operating room. The C-section was uncomplicated.

Dr. Rhea was called at home. The patient was bleeding. She responded to the charge nurse by ordering multiple rounds of uterotonic medication, but the bleeding persisted. Four hours later, the hospitalist (a physician who is employed by a hospital) called for Dr. Rhea to come immediately. As soon as Dr. Rhea saw the patient, she knew they had to go back into surgery. Urgently, Dr. Rhea called for a massive transfusion protocol. The patient was losing blood, and fast.

The patient coded on the operating table and the caregivers started CPR to keep her alive while Dr. Rhea and the hospitalist did an emergency hysterectomy. Scalpel in hand, Dr. Rhea opened the abdomen, while at the same time the patient was being shocked to restart her heart. Dr. Rhea had never experienced anything this severe. Quickly, she called in a gynecologic oncologist to assist. Dr. Rhea knew gynecologic oncologists experience more abnormalities than regular OB-GYNs. Once there, to Dr. Rhea's relief, the older, more experienced oncologist surgeon concurred with everything that was being done.

The patient's status did not improve, and she continued to lose pulse. The intensity of the operating room was suffocating. The staff kept shocking and

DOI: 10.4324/9781003144502-1

performing CPR. This had been going on for over an hour and 20 minutes and Dr. Rhea was worried not enough oxygen was getting to her patient's brain. She put her hand on the patient's aorta and concluded she had expanding retroperitoneal hematoma. Dr. Rhea and an expert surgeon called in to assist did not think they could safely do a hypogastric artery ligation to stop the bleeding. In addition to the already mounting crisis, a massive amount of bloody fluid was coming out of her breathing tube. The patient's life was hanging by threads. The gynecologic oncologist didn't want Dr. Rhea to continue resuscitating. He assured her nothing more could be done; the team of healthcare professionals including physicians, nurses, and technicians had done enough.

Dr. Rhea and the anesthesiologist did not agree. Dr. Rhea responded, "She is still viable." Unwilling to give up hope, they decided to pack her to temporarily stop the bleeding so her family could say goodbye while she was alive as they moved her to the Intensive Care Unit (ICU).

Dr. Rhea met the frightened and anxious family in the family waiting area. She explained every measure they had taken to save her patient's life, but even if the surgery saved her body her mind might be permanently affected.

The patient went to the ICU where her blood count continued to drop. At this point she had received about 140 units of blood. She was too unstable to leave the ICU for surgery, testing, or treatment, so Dr. Rhea called together the gynecologic oncologist, trauma surgeon, and vascular surgeon to convert the ICU into an operating room. They agreed and unpacked her abdomen and performed the gastric artery ligation.

For the first time, the patient's blood count slowly stabilized. From the eyes of the physicians, it had seemed an eternity waiting for some sight of hope, waiting in the darkness of unknowing for some sign of a turnaround. The waiting seemed endless, merciless.

However, that night her right hand and forearm turned black and blue. Over the next week she developed *ischemic necrosis*—tissue death due to loss of blood—in all her extremities. The orthopedic surgeons had to amputate her right forearm, her left fingers, and both her legs below the knee. To Dr. Rhea, it was a continuation of the nightmare: The bleeding under control but new complications beginning. The patient continued to live, while incurring more and more losses. Losses that Dr. Rhea was helpless to stop.

Thankfully, when the patient finally gained consciousness and was extubated, her mind was completely intact. Upon awakening for the first time the patient had no knowledge of the battle for her life that she had gone through or that her limbs had been amputated or that she was unable to be with or hold her baby. No amount of medical training could prepare Dr. Rhea for the emotional trauma before her. Her patient continued to have complications: kidney failure, heart failure, hemorrhaging, an inflamed pelvic hematoma formation, and pneumonia. The patient met her baby for the first time more than a month after the delivery. Dr. Rhea followed her daily for six months and is currently following her weekly rehabilitation.

This was a deeply personal and tragic experience for the patient. What should have been the happy birth of a child turned into a nightmare for the mother that will affect her entire life. She will never physically recover fully from what happened and it will likely be a lifelong struggle to heal her wounds mentally, emotionally, and perhaps spiritually.

The trauma of medicine

However, I wish to turn from the patient to the doctor. I want to talk about the trauma the physicians experienced. Dr. Rhea did her best to save this patient's life and mitigate the cruel, seemingly unavoidable damage. The trauma I am talking about is the emotional trauma experienced by Dr. Rhea. The guilt, shame, anger, fear, anxiety, sadness, depression, despair, and often helplessness that can latch onto a healer doing their best, and how they don't have the teaching or resources to deal with it. The emotional aspects of such an experience go unspoken. Treated as if they don't exist, these emotions become ghostly hauntings of unanswered questions to the soul. All of Dr. Rhea's training told her to push the experience away and move on. But how could she?

Calling on the tenets of depth psychology, it was Jung who proposed: "Real liberation does not come from glossing over or repressing painful states of feeling, but only from experiencing them to the full" (Jung, 1968, para. 587). There would be no peace found in pretense. And there was no training for the present.

***

I studied family systems in my graduate training. We were taught that the child presenting for therapy or that has been brought to therapy is often the strongest member of the family. Often this child will be identified as the child who carries the family pain. I view the climate of medicine and the life of the physician currently in that same light. The family system of managed care, pharmaceuticals, insurance companies, and medical training are the parents who are taking the very life out of our healers, young and old. Who and when will these entities be held responsible for their part of the disheartened, discouraged, and disillusioned physician? Yes, the physician has to learn how to take care of themselves just like a child in an unhealthy family system. The physician has to learn ways of navigating the system in order to survive. The physician has often been identified as the problem in the culture of medicine. I do not agree with this viewpoint.

A witness

Dr. Rhea called me the day after the initial surgery. Her voice was quiet as she stated, "I need you to help me." She belongs to a group of physicians with which I meet, and we already had a therapeutic relationship. She began telling her story, pausing only to gather her tears and catch her breath.

We met and she recounted the trauma of the previous night. She recalled the vast amount of blood on the operating room floor, on the physicians and nurses, and on herself. I could see the paralyzing fear in her eyes and the state of devouring sadness encompassing her soft face. She recounted walking out of the operating room and becoming aware of the horrified faces of her colleagues. She remembered the haunting silence of their looks and their voices. What was their silence saying to her? She remembered the lullaby that was playing in the background suggesting another baby somewhere in the hospital had been born. Lullabies and happy melodies that previously elicited feelings of warmth now seemed especially cruel considering what just happened. Sights and sounds now imprinted themselves terrifyingly into her psyche as she fought an inner desperate demon for her heart not to freeze but to stay open to almost insurmountable pain and anxiety. She left the hospital that early morning unsure of what had just happened. Alone.

That morning when she returned home, she was flooded with sadness and anxiety. As she held her own infant son in her arms, she felt guilt as she wept and began wondering if the newborn baby would ever be held by his mother. She battled within her own mind on why she had the privilege of this moment and her patient did not. She held the unanswerable questions inside of her own body: What had happened? Could she have done anything differently? What would happen? Over and over the questions came like an angry, restless sea pounding against the shoreline. But the pounding was now in her heart, pounding with a silent cold rage, a rage demanding of voice, to words that were unspeakable... Her heart was breaking. Since she was a little girl, she had wanted to be a doctor; the innocence of that call and the oath to do no harm were in conflict with the reality she now faced. The paradox of innocent idealism responding with her heart to a call to help others. Now she would stand alone. No one could take this suffering from her. It was hers. She had stood in the face of tragedy, did everything she knew to do, and yet could not find peace and quietness within her own soul. At this point she was standing between the two worlds of life and death. Here is a critical moment for the physician. She was equipped to respond to the physical obstacles. This is not why she presented in my office. She was here in my presence because she was in great conflict with her feelings. Because of the relentless questioning, the never-ending images that appeared in her mind, her emotions were screaming for relief. Her outer world and inner significance were tumultuous. Would she be able to stand in the presence of such a tragedy and know she did the best she could do? Regardless of the outcome?

I asked Dr. Rhea, "Could you see yourself standing in the operating room? Can you see yourself doing all that you were trained to do, realizing that the outcome is not what you wanted it to be?"

"Yes, I can't get away from it, but I don't know how to respond to it. What else could I have done?" There was silence.

She responded, "I did all I knew to do."

The conflict was to endure regardless of the outcome of the patient's life. This journey was now Dr. Rhea's. The abiding question to be lived was: Could the outer events and the inner response come together in a meaningful way resulting in a sense of wholeness and holiness amid this relentless hell?

The following morning, Dr. Rhea boarded a plane with her family for their long-awaited vacation while her mind and spirit were still in the operating room. She was going on a family vacation which seemed viciously ironic to her now. Dr. Rhea called me from the destination. We spoke often. Sometimes she spoke with emotional flatness and other times stopping to focus and trying to breathe as the emotions were so overwhelming. Her mind spun with questions about what had happened and why. She talked to the patient and the hospital doctors every day on her vacation. She was unable to detach from the experience that was now clawing at her mindful resolutions, living with only the questions and no answers, a place of acute anxiety.

The journey of survival

She came to my office the day she returned home. Dr. Rhea was filled with emotion but no words. The emotional impact was still overwhelming to her brain. She was in survival mode as her amygdala was firing in her unconscious mind letting her know of a constant and abiding threat to her emotional well-being. She had been traumatized. Bessel van der Polk, in *The Body Keeps the Score* states, "Trauma, by definition is unbearable and intolerable" (2014, p. 1). A brilliant young dedicated physician was being forced to go into an unknowable path, alone.

When I am in the presence of such intense and acute pain, I offer more experiential forms of therapy. I was intuitively aware there had to be more than talk therapy to release the emotions that were held prisoner in her body. She had come in on the weekend and we had the entire space for ourselves. I was glad as the vastness of the office was needed for her pain to be expressed.

The daunting images would not be silenced

As she began recounting the story, I could see her body was writhing with energy. I decided to ask her to wait a moment as I left her presence and went to a colleague's office to borrow the punching bag for her. It was big and heavy. She kicked and punched and screamed. She had no words, only guttural instinctive sounds. And yet with every blow, the bag continued to bounce back. It was like her mind. No matter how hard she hit it, it came back. She could not conquer it. She hit and hit and hit. Screaming and crying before surrendering in complete exhaustion. She was traumatized, and I suspect everyone who had been there that day in that operating room had been traumatized as well... We now know that witnessing a trauma has the same impact, sometimes greater, in that the observer often feels helpless to do anything. I wonder about them. Do the images reappear? Does the mind take them back to review the bleeding, the intubations, the manual CPR while being opened? What did they see and hear and touch that sits silently within?

The question of soul

In her physical and emotional exhaustion, she said to me, "I don't know if I want to stay in medicine. I don't know if I want to be a doctor." There was no path for her to follow regarding this confrontation of not knowing. The first 40 years of her life were about knowing logos. The development of her ego. As a physician she was trained to find the source of physical pain, diagnose it, treat it, and bring the problem to a productive end. This development and training are absolutely necessary; however, it is simply not enough to deal with this kind of suffering. There was a question at hand much larger than her ego.

It was a seemingly timeless moment with no answer. Would she stand in the presence of such horror and would she choose what she chose as an innocent child who wanted to help others? Would she respond to her call or would she leave her calling because it was asking too much of her? It is here, I think, that we must provide additional training for physicians' well-being.

"I know I have to go back. I don't know if I can bear it. Seeing the OR... even thinking about it, my heart speeds, hearing the lullaby played in the waiting room took me right back to the hours of the morning of this nightmare. How will I ever be free from it? Will I ever be my normal self again? Can I find any kind of peace in this moment of hell? Will I always be a prisoner of these feelings?" The question was, and is, not how to be free from this. One cannot simply jettison an experience like this and forget about it. The question is how to integrate it without splitting off those feelings and this part of oneself in the process. How do we respond to such an experience to enlarge our life rather than to live a life of diminishment? "The principal aim of psychotherapy is not to transport the patient to an impossible state of happiness in the face of suffering. Life demands for its completion and fulfillment a balance between joy and sorrow" (Jung, 1953, p. 81, para. 185).

Dr. Rhea was wracked with guilt and shame. She reported, "Looking into the eyes of my colleagues, wondering at the shift change that morning, were you there? Did you see? The fear of exposure and judgement. Are they talking about me? Our eyes may or may not meet, when they look away, I wonder, how do they see me? I feel ashamed when I know I did not do what her family wanted me to do... that is, to deliver a healthy baby with a healthy mom. I didn't do that for them."

The invitation to live life differently was at hand. Would she allow the feelings to be identified, felt, expressed, and given meaning? The response to that invitation involved facing her limitations, her humanity, of incorporating those parts of the self she did not yet know, perhaps even parts of herself she was afraid of. She had been properly trained in the dual thinking of medicine. That thinking, however, was now presenting a crisis in her life. Logos was simply not enough. The process of integration had begun, and thankfully, she had a strong support group in her family and the peer support of her partners in her practice. Dr. Rhea stood before a review by the hospital board, and they found no evidence of grievance or error in her actions. She now had begun the process of navigating all that had happened to her. Her muscle memory had been called on and she had responded doing everything she knew to do, which included asking for help. How would she integrate this experience so as not to dissociate leading to post-traumatic stress disorder?

A piece of the puzzle

In the quietness of my home, one evening, I reviewed a conversation that Dr. Rhea and I had three years prior to this experience. I had begun writing this manuscript and often asked the physicians for their responses to the work we were doing. It seems only fitting that I share her earlier statements prior to the above event happening:

> In medicine, in some ways, we are all alone. We alone make critical decisions, bravely command orders. We alone hold the knife. When we witness death, grief, rage, we alone have to hold this with our patients and their families.

> Medical school does not prepare us for this. It cannot. Honestly, no amount of school, or love from a parent or partner can help us through these challenging times and traumatizing encounters. Because each experience is unique and deeply profound in suffering. Only human experience can transform into wisdom. However, there is no system in place to ensure this fragile, transformative process. We need a guide.

> My physician group is lucky to meet with a psychologist on a schedule, every other week. She has taught us ways to communicate with one another, while enlightening ourselves of how we truly feel. There is conflict all around us, because we are in a people-based field. We are forced to be leaders without the skills or formulas in order to lead effectively.

As all physicians, I have personally had minor conflicts with my medical staff, colleagues, and my spouse. Without her, I would still feel bitter and resentful, and ultimately would be working in a toxic work and home environment that eventuates many to burn out and change careers. She has taught us specific formulas that help to identify our feelings, communicate them effectively and request what we need without offense.

As all physicians, I have also had complications, poor patient outcomes including a near patient death despite all efforts and doing everything in my humanly power to save a person's life. Our self-worth is intimately tied to our patients' outcomes. How do we see ourselves then when we have a bad outcome? She has taught me to navigate the abyss of my emotional state during that time.

There must be a system in place for all physicians to process these deeply traumatizing events and rise, rather than stagnate or worse, fall.
Currently, the system in place asks physicians to keep marching forward to the next patient without allowing time to process.

We as physicians need this type of forum where we truly represent ourselves and express our feelings in order to heal ourselves, and then rise to duty.

The uninvited gift of experience

It seemed ironic and eerie that we had this earlier conversation. This experience would ask Dr. Rhea to embody these very words. She would come to live them in the deepest possible way. The experience of her life as a physician would prove to be the teacher; the teacher that would mold and define her was within. The question at hand: How does one bring the inner and outer world together to create a larger whole self, or does one split off and live a life of diminishment? It was the inner world now that was demanding voice. As a therapist, one of the fundamental questions I help patients answer is: "What are the needs of a human being, and how does one go about the reclamation of those needs if they have been ignored?" Many physicians simply do not know what their needs are. Dr. Rhea has been a caregiver her entire life beginning as a child in response to her calling. She could do that job well but struggled when the caregiving was for herself particularly in the emotional arena. She was at a loss. This part of her medical training did not exist.

Thankfully, the group that she joined just out of medical school was mindful of this neglected area for physicians. This teaching is rooted in eros, something desperately missing from today's logos-minded medical society. Eros is defined as the capacity to connect and relate to the emotions of the body and the right side of the brain. These physicians have been taught that their needs are not important. In fact, in medical school they are often taught not to have needs. They work inhumane hours and are often shamed if they present any emotional needs, an attitude that is clearly destructive. It is a dehumanization of the physician and increases not only emotional distress for the physician but can put the patients at risk as well.

When the heart freezes

In the words of Jungian analyst Marion Woodman (1994), "To strive for perfection is to kill love because perfection does not recognize humanity." This was exactly what Dr. Rhea was struggling with. She could not be perfect. She could not make a perfect world that day for her patient. She didn't struggle with the inflation of power. She struggled with the limits of her humanity. The conflict was the loss of perfectionism in the face of intimidation. The heart has to freeze in order to survive. The frozen heart cannot survive and cannot thrive. This is one of the losses of medicine. The loss of humanity and the soul.

Dr. Rhea's story of trauma is just one of the many told to me by physicians. The very coping mechanism they must adopt not only compromises their lives in the medical area but bleeds over into their personal lives. This is often when they show up in my office, and not just because they have had a bad day in the operating or emergency room. They arrive with fear, discouragement, loss, sadness, fighting feelings of inadequacy, anger, guilt, and shame. They come because often they feel despair and know no way to deal with their emotional selves. The trigger may be as simple as a request for their records, a litigation letter, or a statement on social media that was hurtful, criticizing them for not responding in a certain way. Who is there to meet their needs? I contend one great problem at the heart of our broken medical system is the neglect of the physician's emotional and spiritual life.

There is a pervasive belief among physicians that receiving psychological help is a liability in terms of their standing in the profession as they have been taught to tend to the other, but often blinded to their own self-care. Despite research, the culture of medicine accords low priority to physicians' mental health (Ghosh, 2019). A 2018 literature review found the physician suicide rate to be double the average. One doctor in America commits suicide every day—the highest suicide rate of any profession. The physician suicide rate is higher than that of the military. The number of doctor suicides is more than twice that of the general population with 28–40 per 100,000. The rate in the general population is 12.3 per 100,000. These findings were presented at the American Psychiatric Association 2018 annual meeting (Tanwar, 2018). Depression is more common in medical students and residents with 15–30 percent reporting symptoms of depression (of those who are brave enough to report). Where do they find their support? Systemic changes certainly can be helpful, but one has to begin to see the individual needs of these physicians.

The gift of relationship

The recent shootings in El Paso, Texas, triggered Dr. Rhea's trauma as we met in our usual "Group Meeting." (We were in one of the physician's offices, and her partners in the practice were all in attendance.) As a group they had come together in a gathering over their lunch for 90 minutes to learn the Jungian tenets and to hear, see, and support one another. The group once again embraced her and sat quietly in their white coats as they listened intently. One of her partners who had been scheduled for an early morning surgery appeared in the operating room that morning. He had observed her. He saw the final minutes of the life-threatening experience Dr. Rhea had been involved in. In fact, when he saw her, he came and offered assistance just to hold an instrument and give her some sense of not being alone. He had not been there for the whole experience but gave her factual feedback of how he had experienced her professionalism. He had witnessed her being a doctor in the call of duty that any doctor would have wished to avoid. Yet, he slowly told her what he had seen and heard that frightful morning in the operating room. She was grateful someone could see her wholeness while she felt so ravaged. In that moment they shared a gift of relatedness, and I watched as their hearts opened to one another, hearing in a respectful listening manner, inviting their partner to continue to talk about the trauma that had been triggered. The gift? Time was spent listening to the almost unbearable pain that one experiences in the call of service to the healing profession. It is a profession of sacrifice. Under their cold, white coats, deep wounds of both the past and present were being healed... the ingredients? Nothing magic. Time and interest and the ability to identify their needs and their feelings. In the expression of their vulnerability in a safe surrounding called a *temenos* (the Greek word for a sacred, protected space) was the redemption of the call to medicine as one physician was able to hear and hold the emotional pain of the other. Feeling lost and fearful of separation from her very calling, Dr. Rhea faced her acceptance of this journey. A perilous hell is a part of her calling.

The bittersweet call of homecoming

In those moments following this experience Dr. Rhea struggled with a conflict that Jungian analyst James Hollis (2009) refers to as, "Holding a paradox that hums beneath our lives with a rhythm of exile and homecoming." Dr. Rhea was in need of homecoming, being able to come home to herself. Not to do so is a silent invitation to live a life of distraction and superficiality. It is poignant to me that I had been in the presence of a physician who brings new life into the world every day for others, and now I was in the presence of her own rebirth. For rising deep within Dr. Rhea, and all of us who long to grow and change, is a call that emerges... a call to life often in the presence of death. The death of our old understandings and adaptations, the old comfort and compromises.

The birth of meaning

It has been seven months at the time of this writing since Dr. Rhea's experience that was so traumatic. She recently received a request for medical records of this patient.

She called and said, "Mary is going to sue me."

I asked her if she was okay.

She said she was scared and sad.

I said, "Talk to me about you're feeling sad."

"I am sad that I will lose the relationship with her—I have grown close to her and her family. It makes me sad to think I won't know how she is doing or anything about her."

"Yes," I replied. "This is more loss for you. Let yourself feel it."

After a few moments in her feelings, she stated, "I have never been sued before."

"Is this what scares you, the fear of the unknown?"

"Yes."

"Dr. Rhea, the worst-case scenario... they can take away your practice. They can take away your income, but they cannot take away your heart. They cannot take away your soul."

She quietly responded, "I know."

"You must remember the hospital review found no error. Those are the facts." I have found that returning to the facts helps ground physicians when they are emotionally distressed over recent incidents. "You must hold on to what you know to be the truth about you. Those facts can be identified. Those facts represent your truth grounded in your reality. Your suffering comes from the chatter of your ego and what you make up in your own head. Let the made-up stories go, like the clouds floating overhead... you see them, and you let them float away... knowing you are the sky. The thoughts come and go, and the feelings come and go... let them do just that... go. Hold onto the truth, your truth, whatever that is."

Dr. Rhea came to the office the following day and wept. She quietly asked, "How much longer is this going to haunt me?"

I didn't know. But I did know she'd told me she did everything she could do to keep this woman alive. I reminded her of this and asked her if she still believed that. She gently responded, "Yes."

"You have liability insurance, and this may settle out of court, and even if you are not found guilty of any error, she will or could be compensated. Your insurance premiums will go up even though there is no error found. Do you know that? These are the facts."

"Yes," she answered.

"I want you to know this continued pain is something much deeper than what happened in the operating room that day... are you willing to look at the deeper meaning for you?"

"What do you mean?" she asked.

"Who in your history is this woman?"

"I don't understand," she said.

I continued, "As a child, who did you work as hard as you could to make them happy and it was never enough?"

With that question, tears began to roll down Dr. Rhea's soft, but troubled face. "My mother."

"Can you reflect on a memory where you, as a child, experienced the same feelings you are having now as an adult?"

"Yes, my mother was mentally ill, and I have a memory when she was banging pots and pans in the kitchen. It was in the early hours of the morning, and she came and asked me to play the piano and sing to her while she cleaned the kitchen. I had to go to school the next day, but I sat on the kitchen floor and played on my keyboard and sang. No matter what I did, I couldn't make her calm."

"Can you see that memory?" I asked.

"Yes."

"Can you see the child?"

"Yes."

"Can you, the adult you are today, go into that memory in your mind's eye and you the adult walk over to the child sitting on the kitchen floor and call her by name?"

"Yes," she continued to weep.

"Can you tell her you have come for her and she no longer has to keep trying to make her mom well?"

"I never could make her okay. I would go to school the next day and talk to my friends about her. They knew. I hated for them to know, but they were all I had. My dad was gone traveling with his work."

"Yes, you can remember how hard you worked at making your mom okay... and how alone you felt?"

"Yes, and it is like right now with the patient. I have been going to see her everyday trying to make things okay."

"Can you see how you trying to take care of your mom was an impossible job for a child? It is the same now. The feelings are the same. The vulnerable child still lives within your emotional brain. She needs the same protection and love today that she did 30 years ago. You cannot go back and make your mom okay, and you can't go back and make this woman okay. You can go to yourself and see the child within you and you can see she is okay. She needs your love and your protection. If you leave the child in that memory and don't rescue her out of it, the memory itself re-traumatizes her.

But today you have the choice. You must enter the memory, take her out of the memory, and let her feel all of the feelings she felt as a child. You must protect her. Today, that means stop blaming yourself for your patient's suffering. Stand in the face of this tragedy and choose to love yourself and to protect yourself now as a physician instead of second guessing yourself and feeling responsible for another person's well-being. You may have to do this exercise many times before the child is freed from this burden, but this is your task now."

***

Through the application of Jungian thoughts to Dr. Rhea's story, we can see the calling of her task as a physician. This call is engineered by the psyche which may or may not be understood by the ego. We can see that her response to this call took her out of a place of comfort (one might call this "home") of her present knowing. One recognizes that on this particular journey, her task was to respond to the summons of her call, balancing the tightrope of the opposites of life and death, of humanity and the inhumanity of perfectionism. The response to her call, integrating the whole self, would be a gift to her and the world.

Such a passage of unknown territory moving us from one known place to another unknown place is imperative for our maturation and development. This call seeks a response from us, whether it is to our social environment, or from our body, or from a deep spiritual hunger; the call will not be denied. And if it is not responded to consciously, the unconscious will take a life of its own, often showing up in the very places we are seeing the medical climate struggle. Anxiety and depression are perhaps the voice of the unlived life of the physician known consciously. The call asked us to grow, to emerge with new knowledge of both the psyche and the body. According to James Hollis (2009), "This call may not come as an angelic message in a dream, but can manifest as symptoms [such as] boredom, panic, burnout, or depression."

You see, Dr. Rhea was being asked to redeem a value that had been lost or repudiated in childhood experiences and molded even deeper onto her psyche by the demands of her medical environment. As a child, she split herself off from her feelings in efforts to heal and comfort her mother; and now as a physician, she was confronted with that same impulse. But rather than splitting off a part of herself, she was being called to wholeness—to be integrated as a whole physician, not just a logos-driven one. Not to respond to such a call would in fact, invite anxiety attacks, depression, and despair.

The reconciliation of these two parts of herself, logos and eros, underscores the fact that suffering is the requisite for consciousness and recovery of the medical profession. Suffering is humbling. Suffering reminds us of our humanness. Our humanness, our humility, always brings us back to ourselves, to our call. Suffering as an attitude of surrender is a part of life. No one can live without it. In the face of our suffering, we are always invited to a larger call. Again, referencing Hollis (2009), "The addressing of our

suffering will lead us to a life of enlargement rather than diminishment."
Typically, suffering is the beginning of the return to the self, to home.

Homecoming is our goal, and we must realize that homecoming is not out
there but here, in the heart and soul of the matter. Homecoming invites the
healing, the integration of the exiled parts of our personality. For the
physician, this exiled part is most often the feeling function of the personality, and it must be reintegrated. The healing involves a recovery of the
relationship to the soul or psyche, from which our culture, particularly the
medical culture, has lost contact. However, the call of the Self continues to
hum just beneath the surface of our consciousness. Even though we may lose
contact with it, it never loses contact with us.

References

Ghosh, T.S. (2019, February 11). Physician suicide is an occupational hazard [Blog
    post]. *MedPage Today's KevinMD*. Retrieved from https://www.kevinmd.com/
    blog/2019/02/physician-suicide-is-an-occupational-health-crisis.html
Hollis, J. (2009). *What matters most*. New York, NY: Penguin Group.
Jung, C.G. (1953). Psychotherapy and a philosophy of life. In H. Read, M.
    Fordham, G. Adler, & W. McGuire (Eds.), *The collected works of C. G. Jung: Vol.
    16. The practice of psychotherapy*. R.F.C. Hull (Trans.). Princeton, NJ: Princeton
    University Press.
Jung, C.G. (1968). A study in the process of individuation. In H. Read, M. Fordham,
    G. Adler, & W. McGuire (Eds.), *The collected works of C. G. Jung: Vol. 9i.
    Archetypes and the collected unconscious*. R.F.C. Hull (Trans.). Princeton, NJ:
    Princeton University Press.
Remarque, E.M. (1928). *All quiet on the western front*. New York, NY: Random
    House.
Tanwar, D. (2018, May 5). Physicians experience highest suicide rate of any pro-
    fession. Presentation at the American Psychiatric Association.
van der Polk, B. (2014). *The body keeps the score: brain, mind, and body in the healing
    of trauma*. New York, NY: Penguin.
Woodman, M. (1994). *Addiction to perfection: the still unravished bride*. Toronto,
    Canada: Inner City Books.

Chapter 2

The call

The doctor knows—or at least should know—

he did not choose this career by chance.

C.G. Jung, *The Practice of Psychotherapy*

I write from a place of reflection of the physicians' stories over the last 36 years.

As I reviewed what the physicians' needs were, what their needs are, I began to see a glimmer of a pattern in my notes as I excavated the gold from their stories that had been told to me. In that process I was also reflecting upon my own story, which I will share in this chapter with you, the reader, to experience how our stories are similar as human beings, in search of something greater than ourselves. The call, with all its psychological underpinnings, is most often not fully understood as a child, rather simply experienced. The circuitous path of my development as a healer involved the loss of innocence and naivete, experienced as childhood shame. The healing of that shame involved the reclamation of the self and the development of a creative life forming a tapestry. This weaving would involve stories, theirs and mine. Stories of our humanness, our vulnerabilities that science alone cannot bear. The weaving for me began in childhood.

Many of us experience "callings" in our lives. The call emerges from the archetypal realm. It contains the blueprint and seeks expression in the development of one's personality. When such a call is experienced, there is often single mindedness in one's response that compels one to do that thing that gives meaning and brings fulfillment. The call, as I experienced it, began early in my life. Even before I knew there was such a thing as a call, something or someone seemed to call me as a young child. My vulnerabilities found their way through suffering and began to elicit deeper truths, bringing meaning for my own good—possibly for others as well. As I began the process of assimilating my early life with the present, I reflected upon the words of poet Antonio Machado (2003, p. 55): "Traveler, there is no road / you make your own path as you walk." Only now can I look back and sometimes see my path.

DOI: 10.4324/9781003144502-2

Both my original birth trauma and a midlife trauma have served as a calling to me, along with many more along the way, unveiling my path as I have walked forward. I had no choice in the birth trauma, but in the second, the decision was entirely mine. Both events held the same teleological arch, moving what was in the shadow world of the unconscious to the light of the conscious world. This seems paradoxical, we need the experience of both realms to fully exist in this world. As referenced by Carl Jung: "The unconscious is not just evil by nature, it is also the source of the highest good" (Jung, 1985, para. 389).

From a Jungian perspective, I view the call as serving the development of the personality whereby each individual finds his or her path toward a more individuated Self. For me, the way was unclear, often murky, and I was filled with fear and unknowing as the call took me deep into my unconscious, revealing the wounded, inferior parts of my psyche. The alchemist would, of course, teach that this is the place of the *prima materia*, the place that holds the gold.

I grew up hearing an old story about God, in the heavens, crying. The angels were close by and asked God why he was crying. God responded, "Humans break my heart; they cannot receive my love." The angels said, "Let us go to earth and help the humans find you." God replied, "No." God continued to cry, and the angels continued to beg, until one day, God agreed:

> *Okay, you can go to earth to help the humans, but you must remember, when you leave me, you will swim through this river, and when you get on the other side of the river, you will have forgotten everything about me that you have ever known. When that happens, you will be fully human, and you will spend the rest of your life trying to find me again.*

Viewing the river as analogous to the birth canal, we start with spirit and end in matter longing to return to spirit. The beginning of this journey of life—death—life is a pattern but how does one traverse this journey? We are born with a gift related to our call and it is in the suffering of that often unconscious development of the gift that becomes the recovery of the soul in the outer world.

Delivery of a black baby

My mother was nine months pregnant when she began to hemorrhage. My father took her immediately to the local emergency room where the physician on duty told my mother that she needed a blood transfusion. The procedure was initiated, and the physician left the hospital. Shortly thereafter, hives appeared on my mother and, alarmed, my father yelled for the nurse to get the doctor, only to be informed that the doctor had left for the day. The hospital was in a small South Texas town with only one physician.

My father told the nurse that they were transfusing the wrong blood type, and my mother was reacting to the transfusion. He told her that it needed to be stopped. And the nurse replied that she could not stop it, as that meant going against medical orders. My father, who had once studied to become a surgeon, yanked the IV out of my mother, picked her up, put her in their car, and drove her 80 miles to another hospital where Dr. Ricks, one of his former classmates from medical school, was an obstetrician. When they arrived, Dr. Ricks immediately performed a Caesarean section. I was told that when my mother saw me the next day, I was black and blue from the birth trauma and that I wore an oxygen mask for three days until I could breathe properly. Only today, 66 years later, am I coming to understand the meaning of this story and the Jungian significance behind a "black" baby.

A gift of bitter medicine

The color black is experienced as darkness, where no light or orientation is possible. When I reference the color black, I am speaking of the primordial and darkness, of shame, despair, grief, humiliation as well as, gestation, and possible rejuvenation or resurrection. It has to do with death and the cycles of life and death related to instinct and the unconscious. Black holds all possibilities of new life that have not been born yet but remain hidden or undiscovered in the darkness of the unconscious. I can only with reflection begin to understand the inability to breathe properly after the wrong blood (or life force) was given to me. The symbolism of the black, both physical and psychological, the difficulty in breathing (spirit) due to the wrong blood and the colors of black (body), red (libido), and white (spirit). These colors are symbolic of the life-death-life process (Archive for Research into Archetypal Symbolism ARAS, 2010). Later I would come to understand my calling was there, present at my birth, only to be developed throughout my life's task of becoming a healer in the presence of other healers.

When I was five years old, Christmas was a time of excitement and fantasy. I told Santa Claus, who was magical to me, that I wanted a medicine kit for Christmas and a life-sized doll to be my patient, as I wanted to be a doctor. I suppose, even then, I was asking for what I later would come to know as "my medicine," which, to my imagination, now seems to be the Self creating an unconscious longing for the conscious gift that manifested so many years later. My fantasy was that the doll Santa would bring would be close to the same size as me, about three feet tall with green eyes and blonde hair.

On Christmas morning, I flew out of bed, and there, under the tree, was the giant red package with my name on it. It was at least three feet tall, and I knew it had to be her. I ripped off the wrapping paper. My delighted heart knew Santa Claus really did exist; he had listened to me, and now I would have my doll! Then, within that package, I found another package. I did not understand but just remembered thinking that because the doll was so special, Santa must have needed two boxes, so he wrapped them together. Within that second package, however, was another package, and another, and another. With each opening, the loss began to fill my being, as I began to take in the reality that there was no life-sized doll there. My heart sank. My chest felt tight. I heard my father laughing as he encouraged me to keep opening the boxes, which grew smaller and smaller. At last, there was a box about six inches long. Fighting back the tears, I opened the box to discover a small, ceramic, black baby doll (Figure 2.1). This was the first time I was

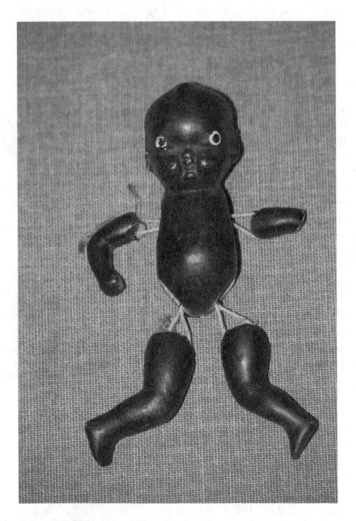

Figure 2.1 Black baby doll.

Source: Content warning: this chapter includes graphic material including racism, white supremacy, and Black trauma.

aware of the psychological shame projected by my father as he associated the color black as inferior.

Though my father's actions seemed cruel, today I understand that his intent was not to hurt. He was simply unconscious. I hated that little black doll. She was not what I wanted, and I hated her for that. Yet, I could not throw away the only gift I had ever received from my father. I heard him laugh and then he broke into a song that he sang often when I begged for a sip of his black coffee: "Oh, you pretty n****r baby, oh you pretty n****r baby, oh you pretty n****r baby, you are black just like your ma." What was I to do? I had no skill in dealing with this feeling. I felt it. It caused tears, but I could not name it. The naming of the feeling was and is important. I only knew it hurt and for some reason I simply felt it. It remained unnamed, unknown, only experienced, with no way to understand it or to make any sense of it. When he stopped singing and saw that I was hurt he said, "Stop that crying and open the rest of your gifts or Santa won't come next year. I was just playing with you, Suz." With that, I obediently stopped crying, pushed my feelings away, and opened my next gift, which was the little red medicine kit I had requested.

The silence of shame

My birth was my first separation from the security of the womb and now I was experiencing the beginning of a second separation. The medicine kit became my prized possession. It was bright red, with the emergency symbol of the white cross on the front of it. It held a bottle of pills of all different colors, a blood pressure cuff, a stethoscope, and a needle for shots. Indeed, it had everything I needed to be a doctor and heal my patients. But who would be my first patient? It was not going to be the life-sized doll I had hoped for, so I figured I would find a willing patient in my kindergarten class.

My good friend Tommy Brown was a willing patient. He was five years old, with brown eyes and neatly combed brown hair. He proudly wore his brown cowboy boots, blue jeans, and his favorite Mickey Mouse t-shirt. At recess we immediately found a space out of the way to serve as my "doctor's office." We took off all our clothes and played doctor. I felt great delight in my newfound profession as a "physician," with my little red medicine kit containing all the medicine I would need—or so I thought. Instead of having to listen to the A-B-Cs of kindergarten, I preferred the experiential form of learning, even at that age. Jung postulated such an experience as this as real learning:

> You can learn a great deal of psychology through studying books, but you will find that this psychology is not very helpful in practical life. A [human] entrusted with the care of souls ought to have a certain wisdom of life which does not consist of words only but chiefly of experience. If such a thing can be taught at all, it must be in the way of personal experience of the human soul. (Jung, 2003)

Little did I know the gods were aligning to teach me one of the most powerful lessons of my life, an experience that would affect my entire life and influence my calling as a psychologist and Jungian analyst.

After school that day, my two older brothers and I were at the kitchen table doing our homework as our mother prepared dinner. We each had our books and were reading as she stood at the kitchen sink. All had gone well that day until my 6-foot-tall dad, the school superintendent, entered the house through the back screen door. His energy was foreign to me. I could see something bad was about to happen. With one hand, he picked up a yardstick from behind the door and with the other, grabbed me and began to whip hard on my legs and buttocks.

I did not understand what I had done to invoke such wrath. What was my father, my hero, doing with his hands I had known only as loving and strong? As my mother and brothers watched in silence, through my tears, I begged, "Why are you mad at me? What have I done? What? What?" Nothing could be worse for me as a child than knowing I had done something but didn't know what. (This would later be my reference point to always wanting to know. The unknowing was/is unbearable. Painful.) After a sustained whipping, the yardstick finally broke in two, and with that, his fury dispelled. Once again, my body was black and blue. This time the very hands that had saved me as a newborn by unplugging the wrong blood transfusion had now been used against me. Silence filled the room. I stood before the king as a broken and shamed waif, an orphan. The psychological abandonment by the parent created what I would later learn to name as the emotion of shame. He told me how disappointed he was in my behavior with Tommy Brown and railed that no daughter of his would act that way again. I knew then that somehow playing doctor was wrong; taking off my clothes and being naked was wrong, so wrong that I needed to be punished for it. This was the end of my childhood innocence. From the previously loving container of my father's arms, I had been sent into exile. No whipping could ever hurt me as much as disappointing my father did. As a five-year-old, I had a horrible feeling, which I had no name for and was helpless to make go away. This incident was never discussed again.

That night, in the darkness of my room, I threw the medicine bag in the trash. I was now doing what had been done to me. Discarding. I had experienced his rage that day which had shamed me. Then my thoughts turned to my doll—not the life-sized one I had hoped for, but the black one. I took her out of the red-painted shoebox in which I had put her, held her, and cried myself to sleep. Returning her to the shoebox again in the morning, I wished I could disappear into the box with her, so I would not have to face my parents, brothers, or anyone at school, where, I was sure, everyone knew how bad I was.

My mother's silence only grew. My brothers taunted me with, "Tommy, Tommy, Tommy," to get whatever it was they wanted from me. I would do anything to hide the shame and despair resulting from my experiment with doctoring. My self-hatred turned into compensation as I tried to be the best student and athlete I could be, unconsciously seeking redemption through my performance that I hoped would please my father, while the innocent, curious, playful child had been sent underground where she stayed for many years to come.

When we moved to a new town six years later, I was relieved and excited that no one would know this awful story about me, only to find that geography did not heal the wound. It was inside of me. I carried shame and anxiety, worrying that I might do something else that would hurt me or the people I loved so deeply. My father's voice rang inside of my head. This was the beginning of me not being able to trust my own authentic self. This was the second part of the separation; the birth trauma was the first and the gift of the black baby and this experience the second. How could I have done something so bad without even knowing what it was? How would I know not to do whatever it was again? It didn't seem bad at the time to play doctor. The loss of innocence, the loss of curiosity, the loss of the safe world needed to be explored.

The gift/curse of coping

As a 17-year-old senior in high school, I had become an accomplished basketball player. Often in the summer I would see my friends going to the lake to waterski, and I would ride my horse to the gym, tie her to the flagpole, and go in and practice. I suppose the unconscious belief was if I could get "good enough," I would never have to feel the emotion of shame again. Please remember, I had no name for this emotion yet—I only felt it—and the only relief I had from it was the performance of both the academic and athletic part of me. I would practice hour upon hour improving my shooting skills. I would end with this daily ritual before going home: I would stand at the free shot line and shoot free shots. I was free to leave and go home only after making 100 in a row. It is interesting to note here that at one time my dad had been a basketball coach, and often at the end of a school day he would come and sit in the bleachers and watch me practice. Now shame had gone underground, and it was showing up again in my conscious world as OCD, an anxiety disorder rooted in perfectionism as a way to deal with my shame. Perfection and shame, both sides of the same coin... both learned and both inhumanely destructive.

A legacy of unfinished business

Looking back, I see how the unfinished business of my parents had been passed down to me. My father was the son of a cattle rancher in Texas and the youngest of eight children. Each child was offered a choice upon graduating from high school: 660 acres of land or college education. My father chose college, as he wanted to be a surgeon. He was a medical student at the University of Kansas when the Great Depression hit, and he chose to leave medical school to help save his father's ranch, which was facing foreclosure. My father taught school, one of the few jobs that produced an income at that time in America. The pay was not enough. They lost the ranch, and my father never returned to medical school. During that time, his father left his mother for another woman. In retrospect, I see that my dream of becoming a doctor and my sexual shame actually belonged to my father. Both of which he never resolved or found peace with. The unfinished business of the parent becomes the business of the child.

My mother was the middle child of five children. Her father was a Baptist minister, and her mother was a homemaker. Her mother provided the family with food, as she was an avid gardener and raised cows and chickens. I often asked my mother how she and my father met, and her response was always the same: "We met in school." That made sense to me, so I never pursued it further.

In 1998, there was a fire in my parents' home, in which my mother had continued to live since my father's death 15 years earlier. My mother and I took on the task of salvaging anything of value remaining in the ashes. During this process, I was completely taken aback to find the red shoebox from my childhood, though I had forgotten what was inside of it. As I lifted the lid, I saw my long-forgotten doll. Parts of her body had been broken, but she was still mostly intact. I sat alone in the ashes on the floor and wept. My little black doll had been hidden away in my red shoebox, in the closet, in my parent's burned house, which mirrored so curiously the multiple boxes that Christmas morning so long ago. Today, she is in a framed box hanging on a wall in my office, symbolizing both beauty and shame holding the duality in its presence.

As I continued to rummage through the ashes, I found a small red journal. I opened it and immediately recognized my mother's writing. The date of the journal would have been in my mother's sixteenth year. About halfway through the journal, I noticed an entry that read: "My favorite teacher is my biology teacher, he is also my basketball coach. He takes me home from practice every day. His name is Mr. Ewing."

I sat stunned, realizing that my father was her teacher! At that time, he was 36, and she was 16. The daughter of a small-town preacher in rural Oklahoma had married her teacher! Was this the root of my father's shame? Was this the source of my mother's silence? Was a naked five-year-old little girl playing doctor their inner demon? Was it their shame that was projected onto me that day when my mother stood silently as my father whipped me with a yardstick? Jung believed,

> The more "impressive" the parents are, and the less they accept their own problems (mostly on the excuse of "sparing the children"), the longer the children will have to suffer from the unlived life of their

parents and the more they will be forced into fulfilling all the things the parents have repressed and kept unconscious. (Jung, 1953, para. 154)

The unfinished business of the parent becomes the business of the child, and so it was. This was to become my medicine. I now look back and recognize that I had been called but to what I did not know.

References

Archive for Research into Archetypal Symbolism (ARAS) (2010). *The book of symbols: Reflections on archetypal images.* Cologne, Germany: Taschen.

Jung, C.G. (1953). Analytical psychology and education: Three lectures. In H. Read, M. Fordham, G. Adler, & W. McGuire (Eds.), *The collected works of C. G. Jung: Vol. 17. The development of personality.* R.F.C. Hull (Trans.). Princeton, NJ: Princeton University Press.

Jung, C.G. (1985). The psychology of the transference. In H. Read, M. Fordham, G. Adler, & W. McGuire (Eds.), *The collected works of C. G. Jung: Vol. 16. The practice of psychotherapy.* R.F.C. Hull (Trans.). Princeton, NJ: Princeton University Press.

Jung, C.G. (2003). *The wisdom of Carl Jung.* E. Hoffman (Ed.). New York, NY: Citadel Press.

Machado, A. (2003). *There is no road.* M.G. Berg & D. Maloney (Trans.). Buffalo, NY: White Pine Press.

Chapter 3

Learning to breathe under water

Nothing that you are is extraneous.

There is nothing about you that doesn't make sense.

Who you are, is not an accident,

and there is nothing sinister lurking in the deep,

waiting to swallow you.

Author unknown

Not knowing creates discomfort for me or anyone in the culture of medicine. In that very thought comes the idea of being under water, unable to breathe or to see where you are going. Jung considers water to be a metaphor or symbol of the unconscious. How does one learn to breathe in an environment that denies the unconscious, that is entirely logos driven? To be born is to be lost. No one arrives with a road map or clear directions on how to get from point A to point B without feeling like we stumble into a great abyss or ocean of unknown territory. Each of us in our own way is breathing or trying to breathe while not yet realizing we are first of all under water. We spend the first half of life trying to breathe into the belief systems that are not yet our own, taught to us by our authority figures. We try to breathe in our cultural blindness, and the compulsive neurological responses often inherited from family childhood. It is the beginning of our psychological growth when we begin to surface and raise our previously unknown periscope above the water level; only then might we see and find pure air.

Chapter 1 helps the reader to see the attitude or orientation of the physician coming from the medical or logos model only, basically that of science presenting a problem that asks the physician or the scientist to solve it, giving little attention to that which is unknowable. Beyond that logos model, Chapter 2 introduces the experiential model, or eros model, with the call I experienced as a child, filled with unconscious meaning taking shape in past events and creating relevance today. This chapter attempts to point out that

DOI: 10.4324/9781003144502-3

neither logos nor eros alone is enough. It is the weaving of these two threads that create the tapestry that transcends both logos and eros. Without both sides, there would be no meaningful life. To bridge the gap or split of the two sides, we must come to accept the reality of irrational inward experience, that of feelings. Emotions cannot be predicted or controlled, but they can be experienced. We must acknowledge that science has an irrational component, an element that is unknown that cannot be measured. It is difficult to measure feeling, but we know that the images produced by an MRI can tell us whether the emotional part of the brain is activated or not. This emotional part of the brain is present in the physician, though often subdued and restricted to the unconscious, and I witness their experiences of this feeling component in those moments that are beyond their intellectual capacity. This is the groundwork of the integration of the healer, recognizing that healing has at its source the unpredictability and unknowability of a mystery in both worlds.

My first dose of fire medicine

Recalling my childhood experience with an angry patriarchal father and a passive obedient mother, I now understand that I had no trusted container. A container or *temenos* is a Greek word meaning a sacred, protected space. Metaphorically, it is what the cocoon is for the caterpillar as it becomes a butterfly. There is no protection or safe place for the gestation or development of a child's personality. It is up to the safe holding by the parents for the development of the child to be curious and explore their development.

When this is the case, where can a child go to be fed? Perhaps my earliest recurring dream as a child points to the teleological way of the psyche: *I am in a five-foot-tall mesquite tree, common in West Texas. It is not a strong tree, as there is little water for the roots. I am five or six, and I am terrified, standing on a limb, holding onto the slim, unstable trunk at the top of the tree. At the bottom of the tree, there are rattlesnakes climbing up toward me.* I awake screaming in terror.

I did not share this dream with anyone until I was 36 years old, when my therapist helped me understand its meaning. After we processed the dream, it never recurred. The dream's symbolic meaning was clear. As a child, I did not have much to hang onto in the outside world. I would cling to the tree for my protection in order to stay alive. Nature would prove to be important to me. I did not see the world as a trusted place, but nature was to be experienced. The snakes were circling me, and their bite would mean certain death. If they were to overtake me, I would surely die, and an antivenom would be necessary to keep me alive. For me, that antidote would come in the form of a horse.

According to J.C. Cooper's *An Illustrated Encyclopedia of Traditional Symbols* (1978), horses have many symbolic meanings. Some of these rang true to me. The horse is a symbol of both life and death. Its instinctual animal nature symbolizes intellect, wisdom, mind, reason, mobility, and dynamic power. The horse can be both masculine and feminine. It represents innocence yet is ridden by heroes. For me, as a means of both movement and containment, the horse was an interesting blend of the opposites. This was where my libido seemed to have gone. I rode every day that I could. The horse came to represent for me a temenos of sorts.

Jung (1968) referred to *temenos* when detailing the importance of imaginative activity as experienced in the unique relationship between analyst and analysand, which creates a sacred circle with its own unique energy field established between them. Could this healing space also be found on a horse's back, between the animal and a child? Could the instinctual energy of the horse be enough to hold the spirit of the child?

While riding my horse, I experienced love and compassion, which dissipated my intense feeling of shame. This experience gave me courage in the face of fear and a sense of self-value that diminished not only my deep anger but also my sense of helplessness. My relationship with my horse served as an antivenom in my psyche as I came to understand my true self as opposed to who my parents seemed to think I was. The wound delivered by my father was healed by nature and reinforced my initial call to be a doctor or healer, though many years would pass before I understood the symbolism of the black doll, the medicine kit, the snakes, and the horse. Although my first calling, in my wish for a doctor's kit, went back into unconsciousness, the symbols of the black baby doll, the medicine kit, the snakes, and the horse were being lived, long before I would understand their meaning. These images later became holy symbols that guided the development of my psyche. In his essay, "On Psychic Energy," Jung wrote about the importance of understanding symbols in psychological development. He referred to the symbol as a "psychological mechanism that transforms energy" (Jung, 1969b, para. 88). Jung claimed that symbols also concretize, in many instances, our inherited archetypes, "the numinous, structural elements of the psyche... [which] possess a certain autonomy and specific energy which enables them to attract, out of the conscious mind, those contents which are best suited for themselves" (1985, para. 344). It is my belief that such archetypes are constellated in my life as symbols that carry the emotional energy needed to sustain life. What I experienced as a child with the implications of the archetypal symbols required time and experience for deeper understanding. Meaning was extrapolated from the emotional content that was/is necessary to continue in the face of the mystery as it continues to unveil. It is the bridging of the two worlds of logos and eros in my life that invites the creativity. This holding of the two opposites is necessary for the enlargement of my life. The interaction of the two provides a greater third.

The space of liminality

Moving from coaching to counseling was a difficult transition. I graduated from college at 21 and told my parents I wanted to be a sports psychologist, which meant I would get a PhD. Upon hearing this declaration, my father promptly called me and insisted I come home for a visit. I knew somehow this would be one of those "we need to talk conversations" in which I wouldn't talk at all but listen to what he had to say. There were no surprises... he stated no one would pay a 24-year-old money to tell them how to live their lives. He continued by stating I needed to get a job and live while going to graduate school and learn what real life was about before pursuing an advanced degree. I agreed there was some wisdom in that conversation and even though I didn't like it, I agreed to get a job coaching while attending graduate school at night and on the weekends. I did this for 12 years. As I reached residency for my doctoral program, I had to decide to go into psychology full time or not. This was a difficult transition for me even though I thought I knew what I wanted to do. I also was facing a crisis in my marriage. I had six miscarriages and now had to decide to choose a permanent end to my childbearing years. I decided I might benefit from counseling.

While in graduate school, trying to find a fit, I met with three different therapists, without success. My first attempt in therapy was to pursue a psychiatrist who on the first visit told me I needed to get a divorce and handed me a prescription for Prozac. The next week I again appeared in his office, to which he asked, "Why are you here?" I replied, "I want to understand what is going on with me." His response, short and terse, "I don't do talk therapy." After that experience, I tried three other therapists each hearing me for a brief moment and then suggesting particular advice on how I could make my life better. If this was what therapy was, I wanted no part of it. I called my department chair and told him I wanted out of the psychology program. These people not only didn't help me, they hurt me. Thankfully he said he would not sign my release until I reported to him I had found a therapist I liked, and if that happened and I still wanted out of the program he would release me. Then I met with a fourth therapist who was an older man. I knew within the first five minutes that this was the kind of therapist I wanted to be, though I could not put my finger on what was different. I just knew he was interested in me and my feelings almost immediately. He was the first person I told about the black baby doll. He was the first person who introduced me to the work of Carl Jung. Over time, he introduced me to Jung's concepts of conscious and unconscious, which opened me to experiential practices of understanding and interpreting my dreams, poetry, art, and the process of visual imagery and active imagination, as I learned the meaning of living a symbolic life.

Marie-Louise von Franz (1964) described active imagination as, "A certain way of meditating imaginatively, by which one may deliberately enter into contact with the unconscious and make a conscious connection with psychic phenomena." I quickly took to this process as a way of visualizing unconscious issues by letting them act themselves out, but not without questioning what occurred. During the first visualization, as my therapist guided me through the process, I opened my eyes and said, "This is bullshit!" He asked me what I saw, and I responded that I saw an opossum playing dead in the middle of a road. He quietly responded, "Isn't that what you are doing, playing dead?" I did not yet know that my self was divided, and I was too afraid to risk not fitting into the collective norm. I was still breathing but had no creative life. I had become frozen to my own ego identity. Frozen due to perfectionism and shame and the fear of being alone or facing rejection. I had become just as frozen as the physicians with whom I would later work.

We continued with my therapy, and I took to active imagination naturally. Six weeks after the first active imagination, I found myself driving home from my therapy session in a thunderstorm and in tears, trying to decide whether I should get a divorce or not. I was so very confused. Suddenly, in my mind's eye, I was aware of the image of a white feminine presence in the car. I wondered if this was a spontaneous active imagination, but at the time I didn't know what that really was. Whatever was happening, I knew to pay attention and pulled the car off the road. I felt an indescribable energy and asked out loud, "Who are you?" In my imagination, a female voice answered, "I am Ishmael," to which I replied, "What do you want?" She simply said, "To love you." A feeling of awe swept over me as I tried to understand how something within me suggested the notion of loving myself.

I hesitated to tell my therapist about this experience for several weeks, as I was fearful that he would not understand or, possibly, that I might be crazy. When I finally did tell him, I was full of questions: Who was Ishmael? My research told me he was the biblical Abraham and Hagar's son, and he had been exiled. Why was Ishmael a woman in my imagination? What did this have to do with me? I pondered the great religions—Judaism, Christianity, Islam, Hinduism, and Buddhism. I was Christian in the sense that I had been introduced to the concept of God through Christianity. As a child, I certainly carried the guilt and shame of the Judeo-Christian fundamentalist teachings and felt that the experience of being cast out included the third great religion of Islam. I certainly understood none of this, except that Ishmael did not ask to be born but was called and then exiled at a very young age, which paralleled my experience. Perhaps this experience was also a part of my calling that I had yet to understand fully.

From the beginning of my work with my therapist, I found myself longing to learn as much about Jung as I could and began to dream about becoming a Jungian analyst. At that time, however, training did not seem to be a realistic possibility, as I had two young children and a practice to run. Instead, I attended workshops with well-known Jungian analysts and contented myself with continuing my work as a psychologist. Significantly, I developed a deep interest and trust in my dream life.

Then teach me

After six miscarriages, I was eight months pregnant with my second child. My obstetrician was diagnosed with a brain tumor and had to refer me to another obstetrician. Up until this time, I had been coaching women's high school basketball while working on my doctorate to become a psychologist. After giving birth to my second daughter, I left coaching, completed graduate school, and began to work full-time as a therapist.

At my last office appointment with this new obstetrician, I felt the need to speak up about something that had been troubling me about his way of communicating. I boldly stated, "You physicians do not know how to talk to or treat women." He was a little put off but asked what I was talking about. I then reported that all he had told me was that the miscarriages were God's way of dealing with a vulnerable pregnancy. I let him know this was not adequate and that something other than that needed to be said. To my surprise and his credit, he simply responded by saying, "Then teach me." My response was to invite him to a women's group I currently offered, suggesting that we could facilitate the group together, with him as the medical director, along with me, the psychologist. Again, I was surprised that he agreed.

After six weeks of co-facilitating the group, this physician said to me, "Suzanne, I am just like these women. All of the stuff you are talking to them about—I am the same as them." This physician was telling me his sense of value was based on his external world, what he could accomplish. He recognized his performance model did not sustain a fulfilled life. His interior life was empty, reflecting the loss of meaning. I agreed with him. He stayed on as a facilitator for the next 23 years.

My work with physicians

He also asked me to come to his medical practice and facilitate the same type of group for the eight physicians practicing with him. This is when I began my work with the physicians in his practice, with whom I have met for 36 years, every Monday for a 90-minute group they refer to as "Suzi group." Although the faces have changed, and there are now women physicians present, I continue to meet with them using the tenets of Jungian psychology. I currently meet with three different physician's groups on a regular basis, as well as meeting with the members individually, both in their offices and mine or wherever there are two chairs and privacy.

Learning to trust

One day, being completely liberated from graduate school, having just received my doctorate three weeks earlier, I rose early and went to see my patient. About midday, I went to the restroom and noticed a drop of blood in my urine. I immediately called my OB-GYN, the physician with whom I had co-directed groups for all those years. I told him about the blood in my urine and asked if I should come in.

He asked me the date of my last pap smear, to which I replied, "Six months ago, and the results were normal." His response was, "It's probably nothing, as you are just starting menopause." Though I felt a bit uneasy, I said, "Okay."

My silence was indicative of my own lack of self-trust, being childlike in my response, giving the physician the full responsibility for my life, inviting him to a God-like position.

A month passed, and I called again to tell him there was blood every time I urinated. His response was the same: "This is how menopause manifests, and there is no need to worry." I hung up, still unsettled. Yet another month passed, and I called one more time, saying I was still bleeding every time I urinated. This time, I added that my grandmother had died of ovarian cancer, and I told him I was worried. He told me I was being neurotic and that I was okay. I hung up the phone, feeling agitated.

The symbolic imagery of the dream

That afternoon I boarded a plane to attend a dream workshop in Boulder, Colorado, conducted by Jungian analyst Clarissa Pinkola Estés. The night before the workshop began, I had the following dream: *I am going to the restroom. I get up to flush and look into the toilet bowl. I see three bloody organs. Then I see Mary, my doctor's nurse, standing in front of me and ask her if I need to call my doctor.*

The dream, in my opinion, was connected to my physical illness as well as a psychic problem. Clearly, there were parts of me that were diseased: The three organs in the commode that were bloody, symbolizing the life force that I was throwing away. This was the unknowing cost of playing dead, unable to take a stand for myself with my physician. The uterus, the symbolic container of my feminine aspect, was losing life along with the ovaries and the fallopian tubes. A passageway of new life was diseased, and in the outer world, I was giving all of my power as a woman to another person (the physician) to guide me, simply because I did not trust my inner life or Self. According to Jung, "the dream, we would say, originates in an unknown part of the psyche and prepares the dreamer for the events of the following day" (1985, para. 5).

I felt alarmed and immediately called my OB-GYN's office and asked to be examined that afternoon. I flew home immediately for the examination, after which my doctor said, "There is a mass; we have to do a biopsy." I think I knew this from the beginning. I simply was unable to trust myself at that time. The following day, I answered the phone at work. It was my OB-GYN. He said, "Suzanne, the biopsy shows a malignancy." I had to sit down to ask him, "Will I live long enough to raise my daughters?" He quietly responded, "I don't know." The silence of the pause that followed, and the uncertainty was almost unbearable. What was being asked of me?

I was sent to a gynecologic oncologist. He examined me and said it was important to determine if the cancer had grown outside the uterine wall. If it had, I knew that meant it had metastasized, so I asked him. He replied that the uterine wall was soft, which I intuited was not good. He ordered a sonogram to be done immediately. I asked the sonographer if the cancer was outside the uterine wall. He replied, "I cannot answer that question, you must talk to your physician." I was already angry at myself for letting this happen, and now I was angry at the sonographer for holding back information that I knew he had. I said, "This is my body, my insurance is paying for this test, and I am not going home until you give me the answer." The sonographer left the room, stating that he would be back. When he returned, he handed me the phone, and I heard my oncologist's voice: "Dr. Hales, this is Dr. —. I want you to go home and try to get some rest. Tomorrow will be a big day for you." I replied that I would and asked him if the mass had grown outside of the uterine wall, as I wanted a direct answer. He responded that it had, without using the word metastasized. The question now was where the cancer was located.

The following morning a radical hysterectomy and lymphadenectomy were performed. When I awoke and asked, my husband told me the cancer had metastasized to the lymph nodes. I was devastated. I believed that if I had metastasized cancer, I would die. Later that day, my OB-GYN came to see me. With tears in his eyes, he said, "I didn't know you were going to have to teach me about this as well," referring to death.

I asked my husband to get my former therapist on the phone as he was teaching in Israel. I was frozen. The only active imagination I could do at that point was to see myself in a casket and my young daughters standing with their father staring at me dead. I was desperate and needed help.

When I spoke to my therapist and told him of the medical results and my belief system, I asked him to help me create a new belief. He replied, "I want you to say to yourself, I am healthy and strong and cancer free." Agitated, I retorted, "How can I say I am healthy and strong and cancer free when they are going to give me radiation, a radiation implant that may kill me, and chemotherapy! You are crazy!" I felt helpless and scared. With a bold tone that I had never heard from him, he said, "I didn't say you have to believe it. I said you have to start saying it. This is how you will create a new belief system. You must get this in your hard drive, meaning making new neural pathways." Frankly, I thought this was psychological bullshit, but I didn't have a better idea, and at least it filled my head with words other than I am afraid I am going to die. So, I began.

The gardener's art

Often, I had heard my patients reference twelve-step meetings. When they were being asked to change and value themselves and were struggling with that, they reported having seen themselves as hopeless and full of shame and disgust. I had heard them repeating phrases like, "fake it until you make it." I needed a new belief system; I just didn't know how to create the software of this new program. But if the twelve-step program worked for them, maybe it would work for me.

I kept hearing the voice of the late Irish poet John O'Donohue:

> May I have the courage today
> To live the life that I would love,
> To postpone my dream no longer,
> but do at last what I came here for
> and waste my heart on fear no more.

I lay in the hospital bed and looked outside of the window. There was a huge oak tree standing mighty and strong, and I said out loud, "The same DNA that is in you is in me. We come from the same source," and in that moment, the oak tree became part of the mantra my therapist had given me. This was the first moment I considered the profound recognition of the presence of the divine in all matter. It was literally in everyone and in everything; we were all connected by energy. I was being asked to reconcile my outer world with my inner one. I was aware I had lived the outer world first, and now I was tasked for the first time to consider body and spirit; human and divine were all one. There is really no duality in life. We are all connected to the one great Source of energy. I recall thinking that if my old belief was learned, I could learn a new one, and in doing so, a new neural pathway could be created. For a half hour a day, I repeated the mantra. It did not matter if I believed it or not; I just had to get the information into my psychological hard drive. Today, I know I was calling upon a Jungian tenet:

> For all our insight, obstinate habits do not disappear until replaced by other habits… no amount of confession and no amount of explaining can make the crooked plant grow straight, but that it must be trained upon the trellis of the norm by the gardener's art. (Jung, 1966, paras. 152, 153)

Could this experience of illness be both good and evil? What would be my fate? Did I have any part in it? Could I be a co-creator or destroyer? What was this asking of me? Could it be that this "illness is in the fullest sense a stage of the individuation process?" (Jung, 1973). Yes, I would come to believe Jung (1984), who said, "Probably in absolute reality there is no such thing as body and mind, but body and mind or soul are the same, the same life, subject to the same laws, and what the body does is happening in the mind."

During my next visit to the oncologist, I was told that my chances of survival were 50/50. If I could live for five years, then perhaps the radiation implant could give me five more years, but I was told that the implant could cause cancer. It did not matter—I needed ten years for my children. I wanted a second opinion, so my oncologist agreed when I said I wanted to visit a cancer center in Houston. The night before I met the second oncologist, I was awakened by my first voice dream. *The voice was bold and masculine. It said, "Suzanne, on your birthday you will know."* I sat up in bed. I looked at my husband. He was asleep. I wondered who had said this to me. I noted that my birthday was two-and-a-half months away. I lay my head on my pillow wondering...

Then there was a loud knock at our hotel room door, which became louder and more insistent. Alarmed, I woke my husband and told him someone was banging on our door. He went to the window and said a large African American man was beating on the door. Again, I wondered if the color black was about my unconscious and what I couldn't see? We sat in silence until the banging stopped. I lay back in the bed and again questioned what this all meant—first, the voice dream, and then the man at the door. I knew it was my psyche trying to tell me something, if only I could bring it to consciousness and find the meaning. My birthday seemed an eternity away. I constantly asked myself, "How do you breathe when you are afraid you are going to die?"

Breathing under water

The next morning, we went to breakfast before meeting with my treatment team. In the restaurant waiting area, I was seated next to a man wearing a military Purple Heart combat medal. Though I am not usually so bold, I asked if I could hold it. I explained that I was about to meet my oncologist and was terrified. Without a word, he kindly put it around my neck letting it fall next to my heart. It was a sacred moment, with no words spoken, only love from one stranger to another.

As I reflected on these experiences, meaning came. I wondered if the voice dream came from God, for coming into contact with the numinous was a mystery no human could understand, only experience. My Self seemed to be telling me I would know about my life or death on my birthday. Only later did I understand the meaning of the dark man banging on the door. He represented my undifferentiated masculine aspect, symbolizing the fear in my psyche. The man with the Purple Heart was a warrior to have received such a medal of honor from the military. The voice dream, the man at the door, and the Purple Heart medal all represented a confrontation between my interior and exterior life. My feeling function was at full throttle, and I understood that I needed to embrace love and courage while preventing fear from overtaking me.

Dark night of the soul

I met with the treatment team, and they were of the same opinion of my oncologist at home, where I began the chemotherapy and radiation the following week. A month later, I had another part of my radiation treatment. I lay on a bed in a sterile isolation room with one small window and was told not to move for the following 24 hours. Clothed in protective suits, the radiation oncologist and his nurse came in with a container holding a radioactive device which would be inserted vaginally. They said they could be in the room for only five minutes, due to the risk of exposure, but would be back in 24 hours to ascertain if I would need another 24 hours of treatment. The physician then inserted the radio-active device into my vagina and used a men's athletic strap to hold it in place. I was stunned and could barely breathe. Though I had books, I could not read. There was a television; I could not watch. I had music; I could not listen. I could not concentrate or focus. I was completely alone. The sensate function of my personality was completely overwhelmed as I lay there wondering if the procedure would give me ten years of life so that I could be there for my two daughters or if the radiation would kill me. Whatever the outcome, I knew I would never be the same. The procedure began at seven o'clock in the morning, and when night came, my fear worsened. Even looking back now, there are no words to describe my encounter with fate that night. Fear of abandonment for my two young daughters and their dad as I wrestled with death images. Fear of annihilation for me as I cried out to God, "Where are you?" I yearned for the comfort of the Holy. This cold, sterile room was directly opposite of my warm embrace of the nature I had grown up with as a child. A dark chasm of nightfall was before me. And I was helpless. Totally, utterly helpless, never before had I felt so alone. The dark night of the soul was at hand with a summons… nothing brought comfort. I could not make it go away whatever it was. I tried to capture the words in my mind I had heard my grandmother recite many times as a child: "Yea, though I walk through the valley of the shadow of death, I will fear no evil for you are with me" (Psalm 23:4). But I did fear. Never had I felt so alone. I was searching out the window of the foreboding darkness for a glimpse of the rising sun… if only I could see the sun.

The symbol of the soul

As the long, treacherous, dark night began to relent, I saw something on the window, though it was not yet light enough to make it out. Then, at daybreak, I could see the window was covered with monarch butterflies—to me, a symbol of soul! I knew I was on some sort of

> The psyche consists essentially of images. It is a series of images in the truest sense, not an accidental juxtaposition or sequence, but a structure that is throughout full of meaning and purpose; it is a "picturing" of vital activities... The material of the body that is ready for life has need of the psyche... in order that its images may live. (Jung, 1969a, para 618)

In that dark night of the soul, when I was alone, unable to read or watch television or even to listen to music and had no direction or understanding, the image had come. I did not have to find the image. The image found me, alone and desperate, in a room of sterility. Just outside of my window was the messenger.

I no longer felt alone. The butterflies seemed to represent new life for me; they are born from the darkness of the closed cocoon. A cocoon that had been as dark as my night had just been. To my relief, the physician came and decided 24 hours of the treatment had been enough; however, because I had been radiated, I was not allowed to be close to my husband or children for another 48 hours. I was completely alienated. I reflected on the exile of Ishmael.

The tension of the opposites of life and death

Six weeks later, on my birthday, a second voice dream came, waking me up with the following words: *"Suzanne, you are cured—completely cured."* I did not tell anyone about this dream—neither my husband nor my therapist, and certainly not my doctor. I was afraid, again, they would think I was crazy. My dreams then became very powerful, perhaps preparing me for the next part of my journey. I was being called to be a Jungian analyst. In 2008, 22 years into my work with physicians, I had the following dream: *I am climbing up a ladder. I get to the top and see a car. Oprah Winfrey is in the driver's seat and Jungian analyst Clarissa Pinkola Estés is in the passenger's seat. I get in the car, and Oprah turns to me and says, "Suzanne, you are about to be deployed," and Estés says, "Your travels will be vast and world-wide."*

I woke from the dream with an inkling of what it might mean. I kept it to myself for weeks, but the dream relentlessly spun in my head. Finally, I called an Episcopal priest, Gene Baker, who had a Jungian orientation and shared the dream with him. He asked me if I was "willing." When I asked, "For what?" he replied, "Willing to become a Jungian analyst." He then queried who the women in the dream were to me, and I replied that Oprah was the most powerful woman in America, and Estés was also a powerful woman and storyteller and Jungian. He again asked if I was willing to become a Jungian analyst, and I responded that I was too afraid not to. He referred me to an analyst who explained the process of applying to the Jung Institute in Zurich. I filled out my application and arrived for selection committee interviews in the summer of 2008. My first interviewer laid my application in his lap and was the first person in my life to say to me, "You belong here." As I was leaving our second interview the following week, he said, "You're not going to be a Jonah, are you?" I replied, "As in Jonah and the whale?" to which he answered, "Yes." I looked at him and said, "Oh, no. Not me." Later, I was informed that I had been accepted to train at the Institute. I began my studies and did not think again about the Jonah comment.

The trickster energy

In 2012, four years into my training, my husband was hospitalized with a life-threatening disease and became septic during an emergency room visit. We were told he had 30 minutes to live. He did not die but instead went into a deep coma. He was in intensive care for five days with an injured heart that had been attacked by a virus, leaving him with a 50 percent level of functioning. We were told he would become weaker over time. Then I knew. Yes, I was a Jonah. I would not finish my training. Jonah is a character in the Bible dealing with the metaphor of waiting and trans-formation. In the story, Jonah is given a holy summons to go to Nineveh. Jonah did not want to go to Nineveh, so he resisted the call and found distractions and tried to run away. In Jonah's story he ran and became a passenger on a boat where he hid. Finally, during a storm threatening to overturn the boat, Jonah recognized that he could not run from God; he surrendered to the moment. He told the truth to his fellow journeymen and cast himself to the deep sea. This is the moment of descent into one's own inner depths. Jonah had been called as I had been. I didn't trust God to take care of my husband and I decided to stay home and not finish my training. I was now separating from my colleagues who had started the training at the same time. They would finish, and I would stay home with only a silent despair as my witness. I reflected on my father's incompletion of medical school and I wondered, was this my fate too? Similar to my father's choice of giving up his dream to help someone else, I was in a place of waiting. For Jonah it was in the belly of the whale who swallowed him up as he jumped overboard. To be swallowed by the whale is a time of going inward, again; I was learning that I don't grow by power, but by descent, by being swallowed. After staying there for three days and nights, Jonah was released. My release involved three years before my emergence of continuing my training at the Jung Institute. I had learned to separate. I had learned to relax to the unknown amidst my fear of never completing the journey, and I had begun to consider my endurance as a way of giving meaning to the journey wherever it took me.

The question of the dream

For the next three years, I continued with my practice and was simply aware I was not finishing my call to become an analyst. Then another life-changing dream came. It was perhaps the final step in my calling. I dreamt the following: *I am at a retreat center in the wilderness of Oklahoma. It is morning, and I walk down the hill to a seven-acre pond fed by a thirty-foot-deep natural spring. On the east side of the pond, I step over two little black snakes. I am aware of them and acknowledge them. Then I walk to the west side of the pond. There I come face to face with an iridescent cobra with green and gold stripes and golden, fiery eyes. Immediately a second cobra appears looking identical to the first one. This cobra is about six inches above the other one. I stand breathless before them. I cannot move. I cannot find words. In my dream I know I am in the presence of a vast mystery.*

Homecoming

I awoke from this dream filled with a combination of awe, fear, and a sense of great mystery. My first thought was about a swollen lymph node I had recently discovered in my neck, which had alarmed me, given my history of cancer. I wondered if these snakes might have some meaning in that regard. Then I reflected on the symbolism of the snake. Snake dreams, according to Jung, usually occur when the conscious mind is deviating from its instinctual basis. I was being cosmically reminded of my call. Though I had dreamt of snakes many times, including the rattlesnake dream of my childhood, they were nothing like the cobras in this dream. Snake medicine is rare. The medicine involves the ability to transmute all poisons, mental, physical, spiritual, or emotional. The image of the snake appears in alchemy. Hermes Trismegistus, the purported father of alchemy, employed the symbology of two snakes intertwining around a sword or rod to represent healing. The snake can be either a masculine or feminine symbol. An understanding of the male and the female within each organism allows a conception of a blending of the two which produces divine energy. This combined energy is often referred to as "fire medicine" (Archive for Research in Archetypal Symbolism, 2010). I reflected on the symbol of snakes in my life, first of the two rattlesnakes climbing the tree (the symbol of life), now the cobras entangled in the caduceus (another life symbol).

Since antiquity, the snake coiled around a rod has been a symbol for the profession of medicine. In Western culture, this image is tied most closely to the cult of Asclepius, the god of medicine in ancient Greek religion and mythology. For modern medicine, the snake symbol represents a human containing spirit.

According to Jung, "The snake symbolizes the numen of the transformative act as well as the transformative substance itself as is particularly clear in alchemy" (1985, para. 676). I took Jung's words to heart and was hopeful something transformational was contained in the appearance of these cobras in my dream. I decided that I was not going to run from the dream of these snakes at the pond but instead run onward to whatever my psyche was asking me to do. My original cancer diagnosis was, certainly, a call to live my life differently. The first half of my life, dominated by performance, was now coming to a halt. What had saved my life as a child was no longer meaningful. Indeed, I had spent the first half of my life focused on my marriage, my family, and my work. I had spent little time developing an interior life. I was tired. In his book, *Words as Eggs,* Jungian analyst Russell Lockhart (1983) writes:

> ... one of the most outstanding features seen in the majority of cancer victims is an extraordinary degree of libidinal investments in an outer object, coupled with a severe denial of something inner.... It has been repeatedly observed that cancer often emerges within six to eighteen months following some major emotional loss, particularly when the individual falls into a "hopeless, helpless" psychology. Such an individual's reason for living frequently is carried by an outer object—be it person, work, possession, goal or idea. When that is lost, a common reaction is loss of will to live. This is fertile for the growth of cancer. Libido turns inward and, unable to find there a compensating value, begins to feed upon the body as an outer object to the psyche.

The unbreakable will of love

With the discovery of the swollen lymph node in my neck, I was frightened and sought treatment, while I searched for the meaning of my numinous cobra dream. I sat with my husband in the office of my trusted oncologist who had treated me during my initial diagnosis of cancer and on through the next 19 years. There I gained my first clue to what the dream might mean. As the oncologist was describing to my husband the surgical procedure for removing the lymph node from my neck, I felt a rush of energy throughout my body, so great that I left the examination room. I was not afraid of the lymph node. I was not afraid of the surgery. I was afraid of the enormous energy I felt in my body, and I did not know what it was or what to do with it. It was as if my body had a language of its own. I could not identify what was happening. I could only experience it.

***

The night before the surgery, I engaged in the process of active imagination, seeking answers for the direction I was being asked to take. The symbolic image of the iridescent snake entered my body symbolizing an opening, transformed in my body in a way we could not see, only experience. The snake was transformed, and the new energy exited through the top of my head in the form of dove feathers (spirit). The dove feathers symbolized the Universal Christ energy that fell in a circle around me, the circle being symbolic of the wholeness of the self. The two energies were united.

Perhaps this was the healing of the energy split that had happened to me as a child. Reclamation of the lost part of myself was at hand. The process would involve the body as the vessel of the journey for the movement of the energy from instinct (snake) to the spiritual (dove). At that moment, there were no answers. I was being asked to trust a journey that I could not see.

The next day, while lying on the gurney waiting in the pre-op room, I read from my phone a poem a friend had sent to me:

> Nothing that you are is extraneous.
> There is nothing about you that doesn't make sense.
> Who you are, is not an accident,
> and there is nothing sinister lurking in the deep,
> waiting to swallow you.
> You are the unbreakable will of love. Embodied.
> Even your monsters have grown weary of their old roles.
> Give them their release.
> Is it not time to renew yourself,
> in the freshness of the dewy morning?
> Even the night you have loved so well, must have its end.
> But the moon, she is still there.
> Now a new day.
> Do not sleep through it. Rise.
> Rise up, with all the other flowers.
>
> (Author unknown)

I wept, and in that moment I knew I would return to my training and to my calling as I recorded in writing the ideas that spontaneously occurred to me: "My work is about healing and beauty; but also it is about ugliness and disease. My life's work is about those who are affected, the healer and the healed, and who heals whom."

With that, I held out my arm for the IV, and I was drawn down into the darkness of sedation. When I awoke, I knew I was being called. I knew I would return to finish my training as an analyst. I found the words of Dag Hammarskjöld (1964) a source of inspiration:

> I do not know Who—or what—put the question. I don't know when it was put. I don't even remember answering. But at some moment I did

answer Yes to Someone—or Something—and from that hour I was certain that existence is meaningful and that, therefore, my life, in self-surrender, had a goal. From that moment I have known what it means "not to look back" and "to take no thought for the morrow.

I know I would continue to work with physicians and their healing. I did not yet know how all the pieces of the puzzle were going to fit together, but I did know that I had to pursue this topic, or I might die.

In times of great uncertainty, I often ruminate on the words of Rainer Maria Rilke (1984), "Be patient toward all that is unresolved in your heart and try to love the questions themselves... Live the questions now. Perhaps you will gradually, without noticing it, live along some distant day into the answer."

The power of witness

As mentioned at the beginning of this book, for the past 36 years, I have counseled many physicians, both individually and in their group practices. This book is about the process I have gone through with them, including beginning a curriculum for medical schools. I have been a witness to their healing as they develop the feeling function in their own lives, which often have become one-sided with the intellect. I have witnessed these physicians become more open to their own suffering, which invites an ability to be present to their patients in a more meaningful way. They become more able to be present with a mind that is quiet, receptive, attentive, and alert rather than focusing exclusively on a particular technique or task to be performed. They report to me that they find themselves listening to their own inner process, as well as to their patients as they indicate to them about the presenting illness, opening possibilities for new insights or intuitions to arise. The physicians with whom I have worked have learned that without saying a word, they can open their hearts and allow their emotion to move as it will.

It is my premise that the healing potential within the patient is opened at the same time it opens within the physician, through the meeting of the deepest selves of both. As Jung says:

> For, twist and turn the matter as we may, the relation between doctor and patient remains a personal one within the impersonal framework of the professional treatment. By no device can the treatment be anything but the product of mutual influence, in which the whole being of the doctor, as well as that of his patient plays its part... For two personalities to meet is like mixing two different substances: if there is any combination at all, both are transformed. (1954, para. 163)

Regarding the healing potential within that space, Jacoby (1984) states:

> Living in the tension of something being revealed or made conscious is the groundwork of integration. Once the mystery of integration is identified, it is imperative that the feeling function is not dismissed. If it is, one may be able to treat the symptom, but one is no longer dealing with the whole human being. Healing is blocked.

Sacred symbols

It seems I have always been immersed in the mystery of life and death. Again, and again, I remember the medicine kit and the black baby doll. I had dug her out of the ashes almost 20 years ago, recovering the symbol of the child. It is her shame that I must now continue to heal.

I must share the last experience I had in my oncologist's office, not as a patient but as a colleague, which somehow ties together all of the threads of my experience. I was talking to him about vulnerability and the need to be open, especially when one is wearing the "white coat." I stood in the presence of this 72-year-old physician and asked him if I could put on his white coat. I wanted him to experience me having the coat on and with my hands in the pockets. I wanted to help him understand how physicians often are not open. That was my ego's agenda that day, but what occurred was much greater, as the gods were there in spite of me. When I asked to put on his coat, "Sure" was his kind response. I put it on, and as he stood before me, he said, "Suzanne, you would make a good doctor." I said something flippant like "I wish I had known that 60 years ago."

Later that night, when I reflected on my physician's words, I began to weep. The scientist had touched the deepest wound of my heart. I had come to bring healing to him, and it was he who brought healing to me. Is this not often the way of the psyche?

My physician had opened me with his words—words that neither of us knew would hold the medicine. I had stood before this competent man, heard his words, and understood the truth of them for the first time. I would have been a good doctor. I am a good doctor. The mystic and the scientist are two sides of the same coin. The medicine was in the medicine bag, and the medicine bag was my life, answering a call that began at my birth as the black baby.

In our encounter, there were no medicine kits, no black babies, no snakes, no horses—just two human beings standing together on a journey of healing, holding a sacred and holy space called a *temenos*. The call was now enacted. The past 66 years had been about understanding I am not what happened to me but rather how I respond to it. What I had disregarded as a child, which seemed a curse at the time, was asking for redemption in greater service not just to myself but to humankind.

> We shall not cease from exploration
> And the end of all our exploring
> Will be to arrive where we started
> And know the place for the first time.

T.S. Eliot

References

Archive for Research in Archetypal Symbolism. (2010). *The book of symbols: Reflections on archetypal images.* Cologne, Germany: Taschen.

Cooper, J.C. (1978). *An illustrated encyclopedia of traditional symbols.* London, England: Thames.

Eliot, T.S. (1971). Burnt norton. *Four Quartets.* Orlando, Florida: Harcourt.

Hammarskjöld, D. (1964). *Markings.* L. Sjöberg & W.H. Auden (Trans.). London, England: Faber.

Jacoby, M. (1984). *The analytic encounter: transference and human relationship.* Toronto, Canada: Inner City Books.

Jung, C.G. (1954). Analytical psychology and education: three lectures. In H. Read, M. Fordham, G. Adler, & W. McGuire (Eds.), *The collected works of C. G. Jung: Vol. 17. The development of personality.* R.F.C. Hull (Trans.). Princeton, NJ: Princeton University Press.

Jung, C.G. (1966). Problems of modern psychotherapy. In H. Read, M. Fordham, G. Adler, & W. McGuire (Eds.), *The collected works of C. G. Jung: Vol. 16. The practice of psychotherapy.* R.F.C. Hull (Trans.). Princeton, NJ: Princeton University Press.

Jung, C.G. (1968). *The collected works of C. G. Jung: Vol.12. Psychology and alchemy.* R.F.C. Hull (Trans.). H. Read, M. Fordham, G. Adler, & W. McGuire (Eds.). Princeton, NJ: Princeton University Press.

Jung, C.G. (1969a). Spirit and life. In H. Read, M. Fordham, G. Adler, & W. McGuire (Eds.), *The collected works of C. G. Jung: Vol. 8. The structure and dynamics of the psyche.* R.F.C. Hull (Trans.). (Princeton, NJ: Princeton University Press. (Original work published 1926).

Jung, C.G. (1969b). On psychic energy. In H. Read, M. Fordham, G. Adler, & W. McGuire (Eds.), *The collected works of C. G. Jung: Vol. 8. The structure and dynamics of the psyche.* R.F.C. Hull (Trans.). Princeton, NJ: Princeton University Press.

Jung, C.G. (1973). *Letters, vol. 1: 1906–1950.* G. Adler, A. Jaffé, & R.F.C. Hull (Trans.). Princeton, NJ: Princeton University Press.

Jung, C.G. (1984). *Dream analysis: Notes of the seminar given in 1928–1930.* W. McGuire. (Ed.). Princeton, NJ: Princeton University Press.

Jung, C.G. (1985). *The collected works of C. G. Jung: Vol. 5. Symbols of transformation.* R.F.C. Hull (Trans.). H. Read, M. Fordham, G. Adler, & W. McGuire (Eds.). Princeton, NJ: Princeton University Press.

Lockhart, R.A. (1983). *Words as eggs*. Dallas, TX: Springer.

O'Donohue, J. (2008). A morning offering. *To bless the space between us: A book of blessings*. New York: Doubleday.

Rilke, R.M. (1984). *Letters to a young poet*. Stephen Mitchell (Trans.). New York: Random House.

von Franz, M.-L. (1964). The process of individuation." In C.G. Jung & M.-L. von Franz (Eds.), *Man and his symbols* (pp. 158–229). London, England: Aldus Books.

Chapter 4

When the heart freezes

Nobody can meddle with fire or poison without being affected in some vulnerable spot; for the true physician does not stand outside his work but is always in the thick of it.

C.G. Jung, *Psychology and Alchemy*

The preceding chapter presented the concept of the call and, specifically, how I have been called a healer in dealing with physicians and was called to write this book. This chapter addresses the wounds of the healer and the associated archetypes when the call of a physician is confronted by the experience of modern Western medicine. It is my contention that this medical model is in need of radical change. As a student of Jung, I am reminded of his teaching that as healers, it is our experience, in the long run, that provides the most powerful learning, rather than what we learn from books:

> You can learn a great deal of psychology through studying books, but you will find that this psychology is not very helpful in practical life. A [person] entrusted with the care of souls ought to have a certain wisdom of life which does not consist of words only, but chiefly experience. Such psychology, as I understand it, is not only a piece of knowledge, but a certain wisdom of life at the same time. If such a thing can be taught at all, it must be in the way of a personal experience of the human soul. Such an experience is possible only when the teaching has a personal character, namely when you are personally taught and not generally. (Jung, 2003)

The path of woundedness

My own personal resources include almost four decades of clinical relationships with physicians, my training as a clinician with a doctorate degree in counseling psychology, and my experiences as a patient under the care of physicians

DOI: 10.4324/9781003144502-4

trained in Western medicine. The accounts I have witnessed or heard in individual and group sessions with Western physicians have further convinced me that there is a need for change in the way they are trained. Significantly, most accounts have a theme illustrating the outcome when training physicians exiles a part of themselves in order to cope with the rigorous training of medical school. One physician expressed this more specifically: "Medical school is when the heart freezes."

The call in preadolescence

According to a recent American Medical Association study, "Approximately 75 percent of physicians feel called to 'help others' during preadolescence. The remaining 25 percent attribute their professional path to the intellect and the desire for money" (AMA, 2017). My particular interest lies in what happens to the heart and psyche when the call at preadolescence comes face-to-face with the realities of medical school, when most students repress their feeling function in order to live in the analytical sterility of the sensate function and intellect. This splitting precludes tending to the heart and leads to logos-dominated one-sidedness in the trainee. As previously stated, the original call comes most often from the rational function of the personality, that of feeling or eros, which is in stark contrast to a training method that requires a strict regime of logic, leaving no space for emotional development and thus causing medical students to be woefully unprepared for the work they will be asked to perform throughout their careers as physicians.

Among the accounts I have personally heard regarding the call in preadolescence to become a physician, an OB/Gyn related the following:

> My father died when I was three. When I would get sick my mom couldn't take me to the clinic as she couldn't afford it. So, she would call the doctor and tell him I was sick, and he would stop at our apartment on his way home from work to help take care of me. He would bring medicine and he would let me listen through his stethoscope. One day, I just knew I wanted to do what he did when I grew up. (Personal Communication, June 2017)

An emergency room physician shared this story of being called at a young age:

> My uncle was a physician, and I used to go with him to the emergency room. I didn't get to go with him to the clinic where he worked during the day, but sometimes on weekends, I would go with him when he was called to treat an emergency. When I saw what he did, I knew I wanted to be a doctor. I never really got to see him actually treat someone, but while I sat at the nurse's

station and waited for him, I would see his patients come and leave.
(Personal Communication, November 16, 2016)

Dismissal of the feeling function

Although the two tender memories documented above reflect the instinctive call to be a healer based on a desire to help people, the following accounts describe the reality when the calling to become a doctor begins to feel like a curse, and the feeling function is often completely dismissed or ignored. One physician recalled,

> *In medical school, we are not taught how to deal with our emotions. During my surgical rotation, I watched a body be opened as an observer and fainted, but I did not the next time when I was given the task of holding the instruments that held the body cavity open. I learned that when I was participating in the surgery I could stay present, but as an observer I could not. It seemed the doing relegated the feelings to exit. This was the time when the heart freezes.* (Personal Communication, February 11, 2017)

In the third year of his fellowship, an intensive care unit pulmonologist shared the following experience:

> *I was working at a large metropolitan hospital. A man was in the ICU and not doing well. I knew he needed a certain medication and he needed it immediately, but the protocol of the hospital was to go through certain procedural steps to get the medicine from the pharmacy downstairs up to us. We didn't have that kind of time. I knew the medicine was available locked up in the medicine cabinet, but I couldn't just go get it. I watched him die because of some sort of stupid policy. I walked to the waiting room, and his wife grabbed me. She started sobbing. I guess she could tell from the look on my face that he had died. I finally told her that her husband was dead. She just kept holding on to me. I just stood there not knowing what to do or say. I finally told her I was sorry and that I had to go. I took her hands from around me, and I went back to the intensive care unit. I think I told one of my colleagues, and then I went to my car and turned the radio on to a heavy metal station and turned the volume up as high as it would go. I lived about 45 minutes away, and I don't remember anything about the trip home. When I got there, I just went inside to the bar and poured myself a drink.* (Personal Communication, May 12, 2016)

As I sat in silence with this brilliant young physician, a tear slowly rolled down his cheek. Neither of us spoke. The silence said it all. The rage was deep within him, and the helplessness was now manifesting in neuroses of anxiety. His need to be seen and heard was paramount. The therapeutic container was the heartbeat for this young man whose life had been called to save others. He was now in the presence of his own limits and those of a system that would allow a person to die by honoring the rules more than life itself. All I could do was be his witness. It was life-giving for him that someone knew what had just happened. It somehow made the experience more real as he talked about it.

This young physician's account reflects the story of the split in medicine. The focus on the rules and logos was costly, and the lack of eros is haunting. He had come to me at the suggestion of his wife to address his social anxiety, his difficulty in dealing with his feelings, and what clearly had been a traumatic experience. His wife was also a physician and a participant in one of the physician groups I facilitate. She recognized the possible dangers of his alcohol consumption and asked him to get help to deal with what he was feeling. He was reluctant to come for counseling as he had been to a psychiatrist at the medical school who was not helpful. This young resident was not trained in dealing with his own emotions, much less the emotions of a distraught woman who had just lost her husband. He could not identify the emotions of sadness, anger, or help-lessness in himself, an ability that is needed when called to offer compas-sion. Instead, he told me he had stood there in front of the wife of the patient who had died feeling, "Like a cold stiff board with nothing to say." He had no tools to help him navigate this human situation and turned his anger inward toward himself in his helplessness. When I asked if he was able to process this experience the next day at the hospital, his response was, "We didn't have time."

The assertion that there was not enough time for this young physician to process his pain illuminates the teaching of Jung (1963) regarding loneliness: "Loneliness does not come from having no people around but from being unable to communicate the things that seem important to oneself, or from holding certain views which others find inadmissible."

When there are no words

The consequence of this inability to communicate is exemplified by an in-tensive care physician's reflection upon his recent experience.

Upon hearing a soft knock, I open the back door to my office and Dr. Michaels enters. I invite him to sit anywhere he likes. He looks around the room and choses the chair closest to the door. I try to make my office as comfortable, warm, and welcoming as possible, but he is uncomfortable here. Simply observing in silence, I reflect on his look of terror and his choice to be close to the exit. I quietly wonder where he had been held hostage or trapped. Words were difficult for him, feelings even harder to express. I asked him, "What is it that brings you to see me?" He says with a quiet hesitation, "I don't know."

This was not the first time I had seen him. In fact, it was the fifth time in the last two years. He presented as highly anxious... he would come for a visit, and a long time would lapse before reappearing. His eyes were black with a harrowing look of fear pulsating from them. He was full of terror as if he was being stalked. This was my first experience of him on the first visit and here again on the fifth visit. Where was he mentally? What was he thinking? His body was here in the room with me, but his essence was far, far away... how could I reach him? I began to ask questions, and immediately I felt the block between us. I must somehow change to become a vessel for him, and I knew I could not continue the route of talk therapy. I needed to move out of the intellect, into the unconscious. I asked if he was willing to move to the art table and try a different approach.

He agreed and we moved to the art table. "Will you imagine the paper that I have rolled out on the table as an artist canvas?"

"Sure," he said.

"Will you paint what is going on inside of you?" I had different mediums of color: paints, crayons, pencils, markers. He chose the colored pencils and began coloring an area about two inches long in the middle of the paper. "Deep blue—that is me." he said, then put the blue pencil down and picked up the orange pencil.

He positioned the orange directly under the blue. I noticed him using both colors, with a deep pressure on the paper. I remained silent, fearful that speaking would stop his progress. I knew there was a deep unconscious process occurring; he would open the silence when he felt ready and safe enough. The next color was green, and he made a wide swath under the first two colors and extended it out past the blue and orange... like a field of grass holding the other two. Still without speaking, Dr. Michaels picked up black, and colored beside the blue and orange, but the green stayed underneath. He put the pencil down, and quietly said, "That is all."

I asked him to tell me about his painting (Figure 4.1). Again, he said, "I am the blue."

"Yes? Tell me about the blue." He was silent, struggling with words.

"It seems deep blue," I prompted him, trying to waylay the frustration building inside him.

It all came out.

"I have a 92-year-old man. He is on dialysis, he is intubated, he has dementia, he is on my floor because his lungs aren't strong enough to provide

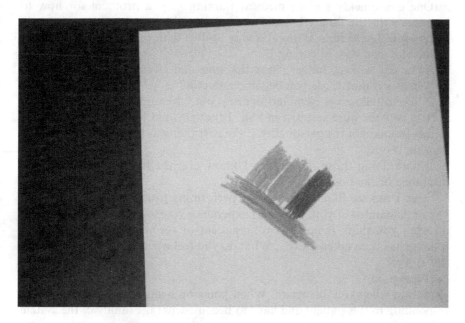

Figure 4.1 Patient drawing.

the oxygen he needs, so we had to intubate him. His family has these expectations that I can wave my arms and cure him. They are not prepared. He is not going to get better. There is no magic here, but his family can't see it. They keep asking me to do anything—everything to keep him alive. He didn't have an advance health directive, so the family makes the decisions."

Dr. Michaels took a breath. "He is not going to get better." He said, slower. "They will move him to some alternative facility to keep him intubated and on dialysis until he dies in six months..."

"Did you tell the family these things?" I asked.

"I told them, but it is like they can't or don't want to hear me."

"Did medical school prepare you for this?"

"You mean as far as the family is concerned? Yeah, they taught us protocol on how to interface with the family..." his eyes lowered, and his voice softened, "It is like I am at a circus... They want me to do all the magic tricks..."

He stopped talking and breathed lightly. I waited for him to continue.

"I do things that I think are crazy like... I catheterize him, and I have to dissociate from myself because I realize I think this is a sick joke to do these things to this man."

(One can quickly see the medical training gave a protocol for how to interface with the family but did not prepare this physician for what was going on inside of him. Without a way to deal with this type of conflict, he dissociates as a way of coping.)

There was an even longer pause this time and I ventured a question.

"What is it that made you become a doctor?"

"I like to take a problem and figure it out," he said.

Here was the pure scientist in him, I thought, but he had to split off the feeling function of the personality... the part that was involved in more than figuring it out.

"I hate doing those things that I know are just for the families or the insurance or the hospital..."

"Yes, I can see that when you are performing tasks that are expected of you or demanded of you, you don't experience yourself as having a choice to do what you think is best for your patient or for you. It is like your autonomy has been taken away... What do you feel when you hear yourself tell this story?"

"I feel used."

"Is that when you dissociate? When you stop being your authentic self in responding to this patient and have to become what the family of the system demands you to be?"

"Yes."

"Do you know why you dissociate?" I asked.

"No... I just know I hate the feelings. I can't' have the feelings."

I referred to the painting, "Are they here in the colors?"

He nodded and pointed, "That is the orange. I think of yellow as anxiety and red as anger that I hate doing this."

"What is the black?"

"Death... his and mine."

"Tell me more."

"I am telling you a part of me dies every time I have to do this." I became aware it isn't the loss of the patient's pulse that was giving him trouble. In fact, as we talked, he saw that he himself identified with the man in feeling abandoned and without choice in what he was doing. (I think this explains the terror in his eyes as he described feeling trapped.) He was as helpless as the comatose man he was caring for—that is where the anger and rage reside.

Dr. Michaels is a brilliant young physician. His wife is also a physician, and I asked him if he ever talked to her about these kinds of issues. He said he did not, and I asked what stopped him from doing so. "Her work is filled with hope... babies being born are about hope... my work is about death... not breathing in the ICU... it's different."

We kept talking. First about the need to name and identify what he was feeling and then to help him discover how he might want to express it. We continued to dialogue regarding the heaviness of the projection of God onto the physician and how it is dangerous to identify with this projection. Dr. Michaels was struggling with his humanity. His inability to stop performing was in direct conflict with his calling as a doctor, and he had no viable tool to help him navigate this emotional turmoil.

"If you can't control the outcome of managing the family's expectations, or the hospitals'," I asked, "What is the alternative?"

He proposed, "I can either quit medicine or blow my head off, but I can't do this anymore."

I certainly think death is a choice for many. I propose that this physician is in need of healing. This physician is caught in a collision of cross purposes, conflicting interests, caught between demands that often conflict with his own values. The healing is not that something different is seen, but that he can learn to see differently. Physicians are called to not hide from the dark side of things, but in fact draw close to the pain of the world and allow it to rapidly change their perspective.

Back to our physician, Dr. Michaels. He drew a picture. A block of blue. A block of orange right under it. A block of black that matches the height and width of the blue and orange. But there is also the green. Several deep broad strokes of green that hold the other colors. When I asked him what the green stood for, he didn't know. When I asked him what green stood for in ordinary life, he responded, "Grass, trees, nature."

Could this be what Carl Jung is saying when he suggests there is more to our psyche than just our logos? Was this the wholeness of life existing within the tragedy, the trauma, the brokenness of this young doctor's spirit? Could he learn to hold the unanswerable questions? Allowing the conflicting tensions to create without splitting a part of himself off? Reflecting quietly on his picture I wondered, "Is the unconscious speaking to Dr. Michaels in an attempt to let him know he holds the capacity for life amidst this agonizing moment of his pondering death. Yes, the green color was underneath the blue, the orange, and the black.

These stories that reflect the lack of communication are exemplified by a family practitioner's reflection upon her medical school experience:

It was my surgery rotation. There was a severely diabetic man who was going in and out of a coma. Eventually gangrene set in his leg. He screamed he wanted to die. Amputation was the only solution to saving his life. I was holding the leg of this large African American man during the operation. The surgeon was amputating the leg. I was holding the limb as it was sawed off into my hands. The next day he screamed over and over that he wanted to die. He eventually went into a final coma. The attending said he would never regain consciousness, but every day when I visited his bedside, he moaned and moaned. He never opened his eyes. I knew he was in pain. I believed the attending physician when he said he would never regain consciousness. One day when I was in his room, I simply turned up the drip until he stopped breathing. (Personal Communication, November 1, 2016)

When asked how he felt, he replied, "You don't feel. They teach you not to feel." The split speaks. Logos is the highest value in medical schools at the expense of eros. The heart freezes in order to survive.

Secrets of medicine

My clinical work is full of male and female physicians without training to deal with their emotional selves in a crisis. The literature of the medical profession illuminates this state of emergency without providing much in the way of a remedy, as evidenced by the immense quantity of articles in the *Journal of the American Medical Association (JAMA)* and other sources of study on the topic. Physicians who once answered a call are now leaving the practice of medicine due to overwhelming stress and disillusionment. In her recent article in *The Washington Post* entitled, "What I've Learned from My Tally of 757 Doctor Suicides," family physician Pamela Wible tracked the etiology of this crisis and described her call to address this sobering reality:

> It began five years ago. I was at a memorial. Another suicide. Our third doctor in eighteen months. Everyone kept whispering, "Why?" [So...] I began writing about why doctors die by suicide and why it's so often hushed up.

After five years of investigating that question, she offered the following statistics and observations:

- High physician suicide rates have been reported since 1858. One hundred years later the root cause remains unaddressed.
- More men than women physicians kill themselves at a ratio of 7 to 1.
- Doctors who appear to be happy and well-adjusted also commit suicide.
- Patient deaths hurt doctors deeply. Even when there is no medical error, doctors may never forgive themselves for losing a patient. Often, the death of a patient seems to be the key factor in pushing them over the edge.
- Malpractice suits can be devastating. Humans make mistakes, yet when doctors make mistakes, they are publicly shamed in court, on TV, and in newspapers and social media.
- Many doctors continue to suffer for the rest of their lives, carrying the memory of having unintentionally harmed someone.

- Assembly-line medicine kills doctors. Brilliant, compassionate people cannot care for complex patients in 15-minute appointments.
- Pressure from insurance companies and government mandates can be crushing to doctors who simply want to focus on helping others.
- Many doctors cite inhumane working conditions in their suicide notes.
- Bullying, hazing, and sleep deprivation increase risk. Medical training is rampant with deplorable conditions such as working nonstop for 24 hours or more. Physicians report hallucinations, life-threatening seizures, depression, and suicidal thoughts due to sleep deprivation. Fatigued doctors have felt responsible for harming patients.
- Blaming doctors increases suicides. Words such as burnout are often employed by medical institutions to shift blame to doctors for their emotional distress while deflecting attention from unsafe working conditions. When doctors are punished with loss of residency positions or hospital privileges for occupationally-induced mental health conditions, they can become even more hopeless and desperate.
- Some physicians develop on-the-job posttraumatic stress disorder. This is especially true in emergency medicine.

In her final statement, Wible wrote,

> Suicide is preventable, but we have to stop with the secrecy and face up to what it is about being a doctor that can be so emotionally difficult... Healers, after all, also need healing.

When facing these types of overwhelming problems, perhaps we can call on the words of the poet Rainer Rilke. Rilke, as a young man, was writing a letter to his old teacher asking how one can deal with the vastness of the world when one feels so inadequate. In a response back to this young man's question, the older teacher retorts:

> How should we be able to forget those ancient myths that are at the beginning of all peoples, the myths about dragons that at the last moment turn into princesses: perhaps all the dragons of our lives are princesses who are only waiting to see us act just once with beauty and courage... Perhaps everything terrible is in its deepest essence something helpless that wants our love. (Rilke, 1984)

I wondered if this could be what Rilke is speaking to us about? Could this be what Carl Jung is saying when he suggests there is more to our psyche than just our logos? Was this the wholeness of life existing within the tragedy, the trauma, the brokenness of this young doctor's spirit? Reflecting quietly on his picture I wondered, "Is the unconscious speaking to Dr. Michaels in an attempt to let him know he holds the capacity for life amidst this agonizing moment of his pondering death? This picture of the opposites of life and death and what is the possible third?

A patient's perspective on the medical profession in America

Let me share my personal experience that demonstrates a patient confronting the medical profession as framed by the above theoretical diagnosis. Due to my family history, I underwent genetic testing which resulted in learning that I have Lynch Syndrome, indicating a higher risk for a cancer diagnosis. Accordingly, my geneticist instructed me to have an annual colonoscopy. Curiously, it occurred to me that I could not remember the name or face of my gastroenterologist, and I actually had to contact the referring physician who provided his name. All I remembered from previous colonoscopies was being met by the nurse and anesthetist who would promptly sedate me. Upon awakening from the procedure, I would go home and later receive a letter telling me how many polyps had been removed. I began to question how I had allowed this to happen. Having previously undergone cancer treatment, why would I entrust my life to a person that I had never met? What was wrong with me? Perhaps another important question was what was wrong with him? I decided to do things differently when I went for my next scheduled appointment to talk to my colon-rectal specialist. Our conversation went as follows.

I told my colon-rectal specialist that I had been thinking back over the years of care he had provided and had realized that I did not know what he looked like, much less the sound of his voice, as I had never spoken with him. I, therefore, asked him a few questions, the first of which was, "When are you planning to retire?" He wondered aloud why I would ask that question. I informed him that I had been given a diagnosis requiring an annual colonoscopy and that if he was going to see my ass every year for as long as I lived, I wanted to see his face. I wanted to know him, and I wanted him to know a thing or two about me, like my name and something about my family. He answered that he had an eight-year-old child and hoped that would suffice as proof of his longevity. I told him it would. Then I asked him if he would have a relationship with me and added that what I was actually asking was, "Would you care for me?" He stepped back and looked puzzled.

I explained to the doctor what I had meant: Would he come to my bedside before the procedure? Would he call me by name? Would he ask me how I am doing and perhaps touch my hand in an effort to connect with me before being rendered unconscious? I assured him I was not looking for a prescription for Xanax or there to ask him out on a date. I made it clear that it was unacceptable to me to place my life in his hands and not know each other. I ended by telling him that if he was willing to do these things in order to have a doctor–patient relationship with me, then I wanted him to be my doctor. He leaned back against the wall, crossed his arms and said, "I can have a relationship with you, Suzanne."

Patient safety

Consider another experience that demonstrates the usefulness of the theoretical design described above. A 60-year-old woman had come to an OB-Gyn asking for a hysterectomy. The choice for such a surgery was made due to the prevailing symptoms of her medical history. There were known obstacles such as her obesity and the scarring from previous surgeries. The discussion led to the decision to attempt the robotic surgical procedure. If that proved unsuccessful then an open incision would be made to remove her uterus. In attempting the robotic surgery, the physician was immediately faced with an abnormal amount of abdominal adhesions. It had been difficult for him to find an entry point into her abdomen. Upon inserting the miniaturized instruments into her abdominal area, there was a scratch on the woman's bowel. It was not a nip. Both the surgeon and his assistant agreed to sew over the scratch, enforcing the bowel just to be safe. Before leaving the site of entry, both surgeons felt the surgical area had been examined adequately and determined there was no patient harm. The surgeon and his assistant decided to open the woman's abdomen area. The uterus was removed, and the woman was sent to recover in the post-surgery unit at the hospital.

Upon making rounds the following morning, the physician was met with the charge nurse telling him his patient was being moved to the intensive care unit due to inadequate urine output. At this point the surgeon was no longer in charge of his patient as the ICU hospitalist now was treating her for a urinary tract infection. The OB-Gyn immediately asked what was happening and had they done a cat scan to check the bowel? He was dismissed by the physician in charge in the ICU. The original physician then asked how long she has been running this high temperature or if it was a malfunction of the measurement tool. At that point, the ICU interventionist said he had not noticed the temperature spike. Ultimately, a few hours later the woman died; due to her religious affiliation, her body was taken immediately to be cremated, not allowing an autopsy to be performed.

The surgeon was tormented with unanswerable questions. What had happened? He wondered, was there a bowel nip that we did not see? He asked himself, "Did I hurry because of the amount of time I had the operating room, knowing the displeasure of the hospital if one takes longer than the room has been reserved? Was this infection from the urinary tract? Was this the result of unseen bowel infarction?"

One year later he received the summons letter from her family's attorney. This, however, is not the point of my story. As he recounted his experience, he said, "I did not know I was experiencing post-traumatic stress until this week when a patient came to see me for her annual checkup. I had delivered her baby the same week as the death of my patient and I had no memory of this woman's delivery. As I reviewed her chart prior to her examination, I was astonished when I realized I had no memory of her delivery."

The means of survival for these physicians is costly. When faced with this type of emotional pain, they not only put themselves in harm's way, but also the patients whose lives they are asked to care for. The care and treatment of the physician is not only a medical crisis but a crisis for the safety of the patients as well. There must be time and process for the deep emotional pain of the physician to be recognized. However, recognition of the pain is not enough. There must be a tending of this vulnerability. This type of experience is often an invitation for the emergence of the soul as logos is simply unable to provide the salve necessary for the healing to occur. A spiritual initiation is often at hand.

A transformational encounter

Jung wisely observed, "We cannot change anything until we accept it. The meeting of two personalities is like the contact of two chemical substances: If there is a reaction, both are transformed" (1933). My initial experience with my colon-rectal specialist clearly demonstrates a lack of relationship between physician and patient. In the US medical model, this is not the exception but rather the rule. Although modern medicine has made significant advances in the treatment of disease, its overly scientific and technological emphasis has neglected the soul. In the process, the healing bond between patient and physician as well as the physician's own sense of self has suffered. The question that begs to be answered is not how we will save this model of medicine, but what will emerge from its ashes.

References

AMA. (2017, March 30). Survey: U.S. physicians overwhelmingly satisfied with career choice. https://www.ama-assn.org/press-center/press-releases/survey-us-physicians-overwhelmingly-satisfied-career-choice

Jung, C.G. (1933). *Modern man in search of a soul*. Orlando, FL: Houghton Mifflin Harcourt Publishing Company.

Jung, C.G. (1963). *Memories, dreams, reflections*. Aniela Jaffé (Ed.). R. Winston & C. Winston (Trans.). New York, NY: Random House.

Jung, C.G. (1968). *The collected works of C. G. Jung: Vol.12. Psychology and alchemy*. R.F.C. Hull (Trans.). H. Read, M. Fordham, G. Adler, & W. McGuire (Eds.). Princeton, NJ: Princeton University Press.

Jung, C.G. (2003). *The wisdom of Carl Jung*. E. Hoffman (Ed.). New York, NY: Citadel Press.

Rilke, R.M. (1984). *Letters to a young poet*. Stephen Mitchell (Trans.). New York: Random House.

Wible, P. (2018, January 13). What I've learned from my tally of 757 doctor suicides. *Washington Post*.

Chapter 5

From ashes to archetypes

The psyche is not of today. Its ancestry goes back many millions of years.
C.G. Jung, *Symbols of Transformation*

In early medicine, the role of the healer was as a medicine man in touch with higher forces, and it often involved enacted rituals. Next came the physicians of ancient Greece, who were priests of the god of healing, Asclepius. This era of healing evolved into medieval medicine, when European physicians began to practice alchemy, involving its contact with the supernatural. In all these approaches was a vital connection between the healer and the person needing healing. After World War II with the arrival of antibiotics, medicine began to focus only on the product and cure, rather than the healing of the person. The days of the visiting physician with a comforting bedside manner disappeared. As the ability to cure disease has come to the forefront, the inability to relate and heal from the heart has become the ailment. A full understanding of Jungian archetypes can benefit the practice of the healer and help relieve the distance between the patient and the doctor.

Archetypal psychology in relation to medical practice

In her 2015 book, *Return of the Divine Sophia*, mystical symbolist Tricia McCannon commented on the source of Jung's interest in archetypes:

> Jung readily admitted that he had first discovered the concept of archetypes in the teachings of the Hellenistic and Gnostic worlds, where spiritual initiates were introduced to the myths, heroes, and archetypes that offered a gateway to understanding the higher realms. Jung's understanding of these spiritual intelligences gives us tools that allow us to reconcile the cold objectivism of modern-day science with the inner yearnings of spiritual faith that bind the universe together. (2015, 421–422)

DOI: 10.4324/9781003144502-5

McCannon's observation raises the question: How will medicine regain this important soulful aspect of healing? What will trigger the world of medicine to understand that psychological insight is just as important as scientific knowledge?

In his book, *Power in the Helping Professions*, Jungian analyst Adolf Guggenbühl-Craig (2015) stated:

Like it or not psychotherapy is related to medicine. The professional and ethical models that guide the physician are in part those of the psychotherapist as well, and the dark sides of the analyst are to a certain extent linked to the medical character of his work. To help the sick and the suffering is the calling of the physician. The Hippocratic oath reads in part: "The regimen I adopt shall be for the benefit of the sick, refraining from all wrongdoing or corruption. I shall regard my life and my art as sacred.

According to Jaffé, Carl Jung separated from Sigmund Freud based on Jung's belief that healing involved the spiritual energies containing archetypes. Freud had opened the door to the psyche's relationship to somatic disturbances while seeing no need for "the soul, the spiritual part of man." After dismissing the soul, he then elevated logos to the status of God (Rosen, 2013).

Late 20th-century self-psychologist Heinz Kohut (1977), aligning with Jung, warned against rigidly held scientific systems which he believed stifled creativity and impeded "The sector of the human spirit that points most meaningfully into the future."

In his article, "The Archetypal Image of the Wounded Healer," psychiatrist C. Jess Groesbeck (1975) echoed the importance of psychological relatedness in the effort to heal. He pointed out that in discussing the psychology of transference, Jung posited that physicians (or other healers) must be willing to be open to the patient's sickness and feel the patient's pain, suffer with the ill individual, and involve themselves in the healing process. Denoting the archetype of the wounded healer, Groesbeck reiterated Jung's claim that physicians must know and participate in their own incurable wounds, as did Asclepius and Chiron in the ancient legends. David H. Rosen (2013) addressed this same need:

To pursue our own healing, we must develop the ability to let go our old patterns, to be open and receptive, to risk the emotionally painful process of change, and to realize that just as nightly dreams regenerate the psyche, fulfilling daydreams and carrying our creative ideas and avocational pursuits can produce meaningful change in personality and ways of living.

In considering contemporary medicine vis-à-vis the archetypes, the physician and the enactment of the healer archetype are of interest. Modern medicine has become so specialized and advanced, the physician is often perceived as God-like and is feared and hated or respected and admired. The patient may come to the physician in a regressed, childish state, filled with fear. In his book *The Analytic Encounter*, Jungian analyst Mario Jacoby noted Jung's postulation that in archetypal situations, an individual perceives and acts according to a basic paradigm that is inherent in him or herself but also present in all of humanity. As the patient with a need enters the encounter with a physician and projects the healer archetype onto him or her, the physician is compelled to respond by projecting the helpless or child archetype onto the patient. In terms of analyst and patient, Jung's feeling was that "The analyst cannot help becoming at times even deeply affected by the patient, and that he had better accept this fact and be as conscious of it as possible" (Jacoby, 1984). Jacoby added to this line of thought:

> Eros is our uniting feeling-link with other people, with nature or with ourselves. Logos is our capacity to separate ourselves from the surrounding world making it into objects in order to recognize it objectively, reflect about it. Any fully developed human relationship needs both principles, the relating and the knowing. (1984, pp. 63–64)

Jacoby also believed that relationship is a human desire. He stated,

> Human relationship itself is a general basic need which seeks objects in order to be fulfilled. We just need other people for our own sake. We even need them as objects for our own psychic growth, for the process of individuation. We need to interrelate with other people in order to constellate our complexes and so become conscious of them—otherwise we escape from real life. (p. 67)

Perhaps Jung framed the necessity for relationship in the best way: "There is no possibility of individuation on the top of Mount Everest where you are sure that nobody will ever bother you. Individuation always means relationship" (Jacoby, 1984). In the physician–patient relationship, the persona and shadow of both are involved, as discussed further in a later chapter.

In her article, "Reflections on Curing and Healing," analytical psychologist Rosemary Gordon (1979) explained that the word "cure" derives from the Latin word *curare*, which means "to take care of" or "to take charge of" and denotes "successful medical treatment." On the other hand, she stated that the term *to heal* is related to the ancient English word *haelen*, which means "to make" or "become whole," to "recover from sickness" and to "get well." Gordon noted that healing is also a process that is closely related to the word *holy*; both *healing* and *holy* derive from a root meaning "wholeness." Gordon emphasized the importance of both curing and healing in analysts' work with patients.

The question of curriculum

As I work with the psyche of the physician, I discern a profound deficit in medical training whereby the care of our physicians is hardly considered. My recommendation is that a medical school curriculum be developed for the students as well as the instructors, along with another curriculum for continuing education units for the practicing physician, with both curriculums emphasizing self-care for the medical practitioner.

These curriculums would include exploring the personal stories of how the participants in the class were called (or not) to become physicians. Another significant step in helping physicians understand themselves would be exploring individual personality typology utilizing the Myers-Briggs Personality Inventory. Although I originally considered using Jung's Word Association Test to help physicians identify their complexes, I came to the conclusion that such an assessment tool would be too time-consuming.

In my work I have found that in place of an assessment tool, the concept of the *imago dei,* as explicated by Jung (1969) quite effectively blended with the work of Harville Hendrix, in his book, *Getting the Love You Want.* I believe the *Imago* exercise found in Hendrix's book (2008, pp. 158–159) to be quite accurate in identifying childhood woundedness (parental complexes) in a much shorter amount of time. In addition, I propose the use of the genogram as advantageous in the service of helping the physician understand the importance of one's ancestral history.

The emotional, physical, social, intellectual, sexual, and spiritual needs of the physician also need to be addressed given their marginalization due to the dominance of the intellect. Guided imagery, active imagination, dreams, myths and fairytales, music, psychodrama, and the arts all provide ways to address the profound imbalance found in the culture of medicine today. Communication skills, boundaries, sexuality, spirituality, trauma, logos and eros, self-care, feelings, needs, suffering, grief, shame and guilt, litigation, structure of the psyche, complexes and archetypes, unconscious beliefs, and creativity are many of the subjects to be taught in order to traverse the world of the psyche using *both* the Conscious Logos and the Unconscious Eros as guides.

From a Jungian perspective, it is important to include avenues for each physician to learn to relate to her or his individual unconscious. An understanding of the psychic structure of the whole including conscious and unconscious as they relate to each other enables the physicians to integrate all aspects of their being for the totality of their personality. Additionally, Jung emphasized the importance of understanding the value inherent in each person's own wounding. "A good half of every treatment that probes at all deeply consists in the doctor's examining himself... in his own hurt that gives a measure of his power to heal. This and nothing else is the meaning of the Greek myth [Chiron], of the wounded physician" (1951, p. 116, para. 239).

Jung also believed that depth psychology can be potentially dangerous because the analyst is vulnerable to becoming infected by the patient's wounds, which, in turn, might reopen his or her own wounds. To avoid this, the analyst (or physician) must have an ongoing relationship with the unconscious; otherwise, he or she might identify with the healer archetype, which leads to an inflated ego. Von Franz concurred with Jung in regards to the wounded healer being an archetype of the Self. Jung understood that "Only the wounded physician heals. The place of the wound is the place of the greatest gift of another" (1963, p. 134).

Part of the healing relationship is identifying the feelings of the patient and the physician. As previously discussed, in American medical training, students are taught to split off the emotional aspect of the personality at the expense of the feeling function. The message is clear that the feeling function has no place in the physician-patient arena. This split must be corrected and made conscious, as it is costly to both the physician and the patient. In the American medical model, the conscious aspect of the personality is held as paramount, which causes the psychic energy of the feeling function to go into the unconscious. As the professional healer is taught to be more God-like, assuming to know what is best for the patient, the archetype becomes split. The physician then assumes the position of an all-knowing god, whereas the patient is placed in the position of being ignorant, powerless, and neurotic. The healer thus puts on a robe of selfless concern and unconsciously asserts his will over the patient, and the patient puts on a robe of compliance while unconsciously resisting the physician's domination and belittlement. The shadow inherent in this tension is unconsciously present in interactions between the physician and the patient. Making this dynamic conscious in the training of physicians is vital.

In the *Practice of Psychotherapy* Jung emphasized the importance of the power exchange between the patient and the physician. If the exchange remains unconscious the doctor will take a more powerful position and the patient will remain child-like. If these positions remain fixed, neither can experience the life force or eros. Can the physician see the woundedness in him or herself? Can the patient find his or her own inner physician? Living in the tension of something being discovered or made conscious is the groundwork of integration. Once the healing power of integration is identified, it is imperative that the feeling function not be dismissed. Without it, the physician may be able to treat the symptom but is no longer dealing with the whole human being.

References

Gordon, R. (1979). Reflections on curing and healing. *Journal of Analytical Psychology*, *24*(3), 207–217. https://doi.org/10.1111/j.1465-5922.1979.00207.x

Groesbeck, J.C. (1975). The archetypal image of the wounded healer. *Journal of Analytical Psychology*, *20*, 122–145. https://doi.org/10.1111/j.1465-5922.1975.00122.x

Guggenbühl-Craig, A. (2015). *Power in the helping professions*. M. Gubitz (Trans.). Dallas, TX: Spring.

Hendrix, H. (2008). *Getting the love you want*. New York, NY: Holt.

Jacoby, M. (1984). *The analytic encounter: Transference and human relationship*. Toronto, Canada: Inner City Books.

Jung, C. G. (1951). *The collected works of C. G. Jung: Vol. 16. The practice of psychotherapy*. R.F.C. Hull, (Trans.). H. Read, M. Fordham, G. Adler, & W. McGuire (Eds.). Princeton, NJ: Princeton University Press.

Jung, C.G. (1963). *Memories, dreams, reflections*. Aniela Jaffé (Ed.) R. Winston & C. Winston (Trans.). New York, NY: Random House.

Kohut, H. (1977). *The restoration of the self*. New York, NY: International University Press.

McCannon, T. (2015). *Return of the Divine Sophia: Healing the earth through the lost wisdom teachings of Jesus, Isis1, and Mary Magdalene*. Rochester, VT: Bear & Company.

Rosen, D.H. (2013, November 22). Modern medicine and the healing process. *The Jung Page*. Retrieved from: http://www.cgjungpage.org/learn/articles/analytical-psychology/101-modern-medicine-and-the-healing-process

Chapter 6

The reclamation of needs

My soul, my soul, where are you? Do you hear me? I speak, I call you, are you there? I have returned, I am here again. I have shaken the dust of all the lands from my feet, and I have come to you, I am with you. After long years of long wandering I have come to you again.

C.G. Jung, The Red Book: Liber Novus

Jung (1982) postulated that the principle of eros is the "Great binder and loosener" of psychology. It is my contention that the marrying of eros and logos through Jung's analytical psychology provides the insight needed to remedy the medical profession's marginalization of eros. Without this work of bringing opposites together and bringing consciousness to the one-sidedness of today's physicians, their suffering will only continue to create psychological havoc in their lives and those of the patients they treat.

Eros, the guiding style of the feminine, is often seen as a balancing force to *Thanatos*, the death drive, and we are in the throes of such a death as we experience so many doctors and other practitioners leaving because of pressure. The radical decline of eros in medicine became painfully obvious after World War II, when the industrialization and assembly-line culture of business had taken hold in America. Obsessed with increasing productivity and reducing costs resulted in a frenzy of capitalism by the 1980s, when medicine turned from being a care-driven service entity to an economic, prosperity-based industry. Hungry for power and wealth, a new corporate model of healthcare for profit was created. Insurance and pharmaceutical companies readily joined the movement for the possibility of using medicine as an avenue to increase profit. Capitalism had entered the healthcare field, and soon, doctors were put on the assembly lines of patient care. With logos-driven principles now fully in charge of the American health system, physicians felt devalued and degraded, resulting in one-sided medicine. Eros was silenced.

If we are to bring life and vitality back to the field of medicine, there must be an attempt to bring the feminine into the arena to counter this masculine, logos-dominated culture. Jung understood the psyche to be a relatively

DOI: 10.4324/9781003144502-6

closed system that manifests energy in the life process. Within the system, psychic energy flows between two opposites, which serve as a kind of regulating system. When the opposites are relatively balanced, a feeling of equilibrium is experienced. This is the process of progression in which one is able to meet the demands of outer life. The feminine represents a style of being and relating as expressed through eros. To access eros, a physician's needs must be acknowledged and honored. Jay, an internal medicine physician, commented on this necessity in a conversation we shared:

> *It is interesting you are writing on healing the healer. I am a healer and I need healing. But I don't know how to do what you are talking about. I do not know where to begin. I do not know what is missing.* (Personal Communication, January 8, 2016)

I perceived this physician as acknowledging that he was in danger of losing his soul and had no way to deal with his dilemma. Recognizing his desire to identify his needs is the first step to healing through eros.

A most fundamental question with beginnings rooted in eros is the following: "What are the needs of a human being, and how does one go about the reclamation of those needs if they have been ignored?" Many physicians simply do not know what their needs are. Historically they have been taught that their needs are not important. In fact, as previously discussed, in medical school they are often taught not to have needs. They work inhumane hours and are often shamed if they present any emotional needs, which is also inhumane. A now-retired physician recalled his first year as a medical student:

> *Beginning medical students need an orientation to prepare them for the extremely competitive environment they are walking into. Medical school is full of top students. Being "number one in the class," takes on a new meaning. We were all smart, yet we were all screamed at and humiliated. I remember watching a baby die in another resident's arms and the attending physician yelling, "How many babies are you going to have to kill?" Nobody gets over that. Nobody. I was terrorized and filled with shame for him and for me. I wished there had been a place to talk about these experiences but there wasn't. We all seemed to carry on in silence about such things. Saying it out loud would have been seen as weakness. Only the world of thinking and facts seemed acceptable. Why were our needs pushed aside? It was all so punitive. The words punitive and healer don't seem to go together.* (Personal Communication, December 3, 2017)

The story above is just one of many on the same theme told to me by physicians. The very coping mechanism they must adopt not only compromises their lives in the medical area but bleeds over into their personal lives. That is when they show up in my office, and not just because they have had a bad day in the operating or emergency room. They arrive with neurosis. The trigger may be as simple as a request for their records, a litigation letter, or a statement that was hurtful, criticizing them for not responding in a certain way. Who is there to meet their needs? The problem at the heart of our broken medical system is the neglect of the physician's emotional and spiritual life.

In this vein, I am reminded that physicians have repeatedly said they need someone to help them learn to identify and meet their inner needs and to advocate for a wider recognition of these needs. I currently have two physicians who drive over 100 miles to see me for therapeutic intervention. They pay cash because they do not want a paper trail, because in the medical culture, engaging in psychological services can be used against them. Sadly, when they are credentialed, they are asked to disclose if they have ever been treated for depression, anxiety, or mental illness and if they are taking any psychotropic medications. If they tell the truth, they come under suspicion. This is a no-win situation for the physician, for the patient, and the medical community. Why do we accommodate such inhumane behavior by medical licensing boards? The pervasive belief among physicians that receiving psychological help is a liability in terms of their standing in the profession is substantiated by a consensus study of 15 experts in the field of preventing physician suicide. These experts concluded,

> The culture of medicine accords low priority to physician mental health despite evidence of untreated mood disorders and an increased burden of suicide. Barriers to physicians' seeking help are often punitive, including discrimination in medical licensing, hospital privileges, and professional advancement. This consensus statement recommends transforming professional attitudes and changing institutional policies to encourage physicians to seek help. As barriers are removed and physicians confront depression and suicidality in their peers, they are more likely to recognize and treat these conditions in patients, including colleagues and medical students. (Center et al., 2003, p. 289)

During my sessions with physicians, they reported feeling limited in their choice of friends in order to hide neuroses. Due to shame and fear, they often suppress the need for relationship, resulting in excessively private and isolated lives. Most physicians associate with other physicians exclusively, thereby limiting associations that would fulfill their need for friendship.

On the topic of emotional needs, during a group session, one physician expressed lack of understanding:

> *I don't know how to take care of that part of myself. I don't know what you are talking about, really. I thought my needs were to provide safety*

and security for my family and to develop the intellectual needs of my sons. I am dependent on what other people think of me, and I seek their approval to be okay. You are calling that codependency. Can you really teach us how to meet our own needs?(Personal Communication, April 23, 2017)

This interaction proved to be a pivotal moment in my professional career. As an outsider, which is the orphan's archetype, I was trusted by this group of physicians to enter into the closed, exclusive world of Western medicine. Again, the constellation of the archetype had invited me into the presence of the king to reveal the secret of the archetype of the dumbling, which reflected the gold of their unconscious shadow.

Jung stated,

> Loss of soul amounts to a tearing loose of part of one's nature; it is the disappearance and emancipation of a complex, which thereupon becomes a tyrannical usurper of consciousness, oppressing the whole man. It throws him off course and drives him to actions whose blind one-sidedness inevitably leads to self-destruction. (1982, p. 226, para. 384)

This effect is demonstrated by the following experience with Mark, a neurologist, two years out of residency and recently diagnosed with muscular dystrophy. He was facing an overwhelming amount of financial debt in the form of student loans and medical bills as well as the possibility of losing his new practice due to policies based on algorithms of eligibility created by insurance companies that determine his ability to make a living in his profession, all the while fighting the physical manifestations of his disease.

Upon arrival, Mark would not come through the front door of my practice for fear of repercussions related to his physical limitations if observed by his patients or others in the community. He entered through the back entrance to my office. When I asked what brought him to our session, relying on the one-sidedness of logos, he stated facts regarding the needs, responsibilities, expectations, and desires of others. When asked about his own needs, the only one he could relate was the need to walk. His unconsciousness of his basic needs such as love, acceptance, and medical, spiritual, and emotional care reflects the oppression of the whole man, leading to self-destruction as Jung taught. Only after his spouse expressed her experience of him as building a wall around himself and shutting her and the children out, did Mark stop to consider his own emotional needs. He had completely isolated himself due to the shame and fear of his own vulnerability.

Mark's self-hatred regarding the possibility of passing his genetic disease on to his children had created a wall of fear-based shame and isolation. He first isolated himself, then increased his isolation by shutting out those he most loved, his wife and children. Applying the research documented in this book, I then demonstrated acceptance of my own vulnerability by communicating our shared experience of the possibility of passing a genetic weakness onto one's children—in my case, cancer. Creating a bridge of commonality allowed him to open up and recognize his needs.

Jung said that eros can be experienced in the form of a woman, as representative as soul for oneself, or in the form of the divine child (Owens, 2015, p. 5). Both of these forms of eros are ways that physicians can learn to care for themselves. By bringing awareness to the physician's needs through eros, Mark and I were able to join in the temenos. Mark's response to our session was a softening of his spirit and demeanor as well as a new openness to discovering and meeting his own emotional needs, thereby liberating the "whole man" to accept his humanity and receive the love of his family.

In his book, *The Soul's Code: In Search of Character and Calling* (1996), Hillman purported that each human being is born with an energy or life force or spark within. I define this spark, as does Jung, as the libido; it is the life force that drives us to create, to seek knowledge, and to grow. Hillman also suggested that if we can identify and work with that spark, it will be our daemon; ignore it, and it will become our demon.

A relationship to the self, to the other, and to the divine is necessary to a life of individuation. This spark is at the root of all relationships. The life force within has needs that must be addressed. Meeting those needs pulls a human being toward growth and development. Each day as an analyst, I witness the devastation wrought by ignoring the unidentified needs of the spark and physicians' inability to care for the self. As I contemplate the mass shooting of schoolchildren in America, I wonder, *Is this not the demon that Hillman was suggesting? And how are we responsible creating this epidemic of children killing children, or physicians killing themselves or their patients?* I suggest that the answer lies in the relational aspect of the culture, whether it be the family, the school system, the medical school, or the political arena of corporate America. Where there is no relationship, there is power or violence. In Figure 6.1, Abraham Maslow's hierarchy of needs demonstrates the process one must complete in order to care adequately for the self. The ability to care for the self is required before one can effectively care for another.

Another method to help physicians identify needs is to employ their belief system that views a child having needs as acceptable in contrast to their perception of adult needs. When working with clients who are unaware of or repressing their needs, I ask them how they might care for a child. They are usually swift to list ways to meet a child's need to feel loved, safe, or cared for. I then help them see how their own needs are reflected in the needs of the child.

In the therapy process, this would be the time I would introduce the archetype of the child and the never-ending need for growth to obtain individuation. In his essay, "On the Psychology of the Child Archetype," Jung stated, "In every adult there lurks a child—an eternal child—something that is always becoming, is never completed, and calls for the unceasing care,

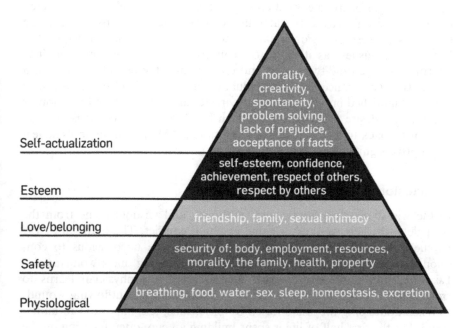

Figure 6.1 Maslow's hierarchy of needs.

attention and education. This is the part of the personality which wants to develop and become whole" (1968, pp. 169–170, para. 286). The teleological orientation promotes the view that human existence has an ongoing development. One of the tenets of depth psychology that I find so helpful is that of the soul's curiosity, unceasing pursuit of knowledge, and desire to grow. This concept often comes as a surprise to the physicians I see, as they frequently propose that, as adults, they have already completed their developmental tasks in life.

Jung's direction was that human beings proceed toward a goal through life cycles that are based on archetypal energies, with each phase in life requiring a new attitude, a renewed orientation and an adjustment of oneself. Often, the midlife passage asks the physician to move from the external values of his life toward an interiority, orienting, perhaps for the first time, toward death. Jung stated that "life is teleology *par excellence*; it is the intrinsic striving towards a goal, and the living organism is a system of directed aims which seek to fulfil themselves. The end of every process is its goal" (1969, p. 406, para. 798). Jung expressed a deeply religious orientation when he stated, "The decisive question for man is: Is he related to something infinite or not? This is the telling question of his life" (1963, 325).

From incorporating Jungian psychology into my practice, I have seen that eros, in its broadest working definition, is the unconscious desire to relate or connect. Logos is eros's eternal compensatory opposite. What is connected or related through eros is separated into consciousness by logos. Logos is the conscious process of logic and articulation but is also that principle that births consciousness as it extricates concepts from the unconscious. The interplay between the two, logos and eros, creates the psychodynamic of a dance. In such a dance, one's individual distinctiveness and personal power are not diminished but are enhanced by relatedness. This desire for union or oneness is a desire to reunite that which has been separated. It is eros we must bring back to medicine, for as Jung stated, "All uniting symbols have a redemptive significance" (1969, p. 168, para. 285).

Conclusion

In the wisest people I know, their authority and wisdom come from the struggle with their wounds or some essential conflict. The material of the psyche seemingly has been able to move from the unconscious to consciousness through conflict and hardship, bringing hard-won insight. Likewise, in the Western medical model, either the physician learns to transform the pain within themselves, or it becomes an outflowing wound.

When addressing the issues raised by physicians, it is important to understand that the first half of life is spent building an ego, often focusing on the logos, or the intellect or rational mind. As mentioned in the previous chapter, the intellectual needs of the medical student receive attention, but they are forced to split off their emotional needs. One might even say those needs are denigrated. This rift between logos and eros becomes a gaping maw as training physicians become externally focused without tending to their inner world and inherent needs. This situation creates a fertile ground for a psychological crisis to grow. For individuation to occur, the psyche must continually endeavor to bring two halves of being together to form a whole.

The following experiences are those of physicians who, in fact, have learned to view their needs through a Jungian lens. Like all of us, they have been deeply wounded in the eros–logos split; yet, as Woodman (1969) said,

> There is an evolution going on here and we have no idea where it is going... We are the people of the transition, and we have heavy work to do... Our imagery, dreams, instincts, and holy energy are carrying us toward a new kind of wholeness in which the old paradigm based on power gives way to one of love and the feminine and the masculine energies will find new balance.

We are moving toward a new feminine consciousness and a new masculine consciousness. The nature of the balance of the masculine and feminine is reflected in the account of a female physician married to a male physician. In desperation, the couple came to see me when she realized her husband was not the "magical other," who would meet all of her needs. She thought it was his responsibility to make her happy:

I thought that was love. He was handsome, smart, romantic, and loved so many of the same things I did. We were so happy in the beginning. We met in medical school and married after finishing residency. I specialized in neurology and he became a pediatrician. I thought we had it all—money, possessions— all the things money can buy. When things changed, he would come home late from work, eat dinner, and watch TV until bedtime. I would try talking to him and would initiate lovemaking. He would often become impatient. I did everything I could think of to regain his interest. This isn't supposed to happen, not to us anyway. (Personal Communication, May 2016)

She looked at me and stated that she could not believe they were in a therapist's office, and she started to cry. She expressed passive suicidal ideation. Neither of them knew what was causing pain in their relationship. She revealed that her parents had a long-term sustained marriage, with her father as the "emotional" one and her mother as the disciplinarian. She reported that they showed little affection to one another and did not fight or talk about their feelings. She and her siblings were taught not to express their feelings and to be thankful for what they had. Her father's work made him somewhat of an absent father, while her mother remained at home taking care of the house and children.

Her husband reported that his parents divorced when he was 12 years old, after which he lived with his mother. He described her as broken-hearted, and he and his sibling seemed to be in charge of making her happy. Being unable to satisfy his mother, he felt resentment. He spent time with his father as often as he could. His father was an extremely successful businessman who always seemed to have women around. He felt proud of his father yet ashamed of him in some way.

After long-term therapy with this female physician, she was able to take back her animus projection on her husband, realizing that it was not his job to make her happy. Likewise, her husband had to come to the understanding that he had spent his childhood unsuccessfully taking care of his mother's needs and how this had manifested in their marriage. He, too, had to pull back his anima projection. This is painful work. It means leaving the magical, idealized projection of romantic love and engaging in developing the maturity to accept the otherness of the partner. This can only be accomplished when they individually integrate into themselves what they have previously projected. Their mutual experience as physicians, with training and work environments that prohibited having needs, only reinforced their lack of understanding with regard to their needs and getting those needs met.

A healthy model

The following physician's story is filled with an urgency to have his needs met, and it is clear how conflicted and desperate he was when he finally called for help. The physician was an ongoing client who had called my office midday to see if I had any cancellations that same day. He was told I could see him at 6:00 PM, but he demurred, stating that he knew I "needed to get home." He told my staff that the issue he wanted to discuss could wait until our regularly scheduled session the following week. Then, around 4:00 PM, he called again to see if he could still come and was told that the 6:00 PM appointment was still available. When he arrived, his first words were, "I need to be seen, I need to be heard, I need to be validated, I need to be loved—that is why I'm here" (Personal Communication, January 2018). He knew from our previous physician-group experiences that he could express himself in this way. He explained that he had received a letter from a former patient's attorney informing him of a lawsuit against him stemming from his patient's ureter being cut during surgery. In reviewing the case, he told me he had looked closely at the post-op images with his treatment team that day and that he had been careful to do everything required surgically. The next day he had discharged the patient. Clearly, unexpected complications arose.

For the purpose of this book, the outcome of this lawsuit is irrelevant. The emotional process of this physician is what matters. Often, when physicians receive such a letter, their well-being is threatened, and their recourse is to hide. Reaching out for protection, they contact their attorneys, who will advise them not to talk to anyone regarding their case. I assert that it is necessary for physicians in this situation to be discerning when they choose to speak with someone about the case, but the antidote for their anxiety is exactly what this doctor did by reaching out to a safe person, his analyst, to explain what was happening in his professional arena. It is telling that even in trying to make an appointment to see me, he was initially reticent to take the time offered earlier in the day. Notably, somewhere inside of him was the discomfort of having needs, and the strong inner pressure to find a harbor for his needs won out by the end of that afternoon. In the end, instead of hiding his loneliness, despair, fear, and shame, he was able to accept that he had the safe container of my office in which he could express his feeling so that his needs might be met. This ability to accept and meet his own needs allows him to be fully present in relationships, professionally and personally.

The medical culture has encouraged a system in which physician needs are marginalized, leaving them with little choice but to suppress them and suffer quietly. Viewed with an analytical perspective, the accounts related in this book reflect the vacuum left either by parental complex material or the introjected messages from medical school. The physicians who explored the lack of attention to their feelings all came to understand that their longing to fill that vacuum is a healthy, human need. In speaking their respective truths, they were able to move toward wholeness and the integration of their deepest selves.

The first half of life is spent building an ego, often at the expense of many other needs. Certainly, for the medical student, their intellectual needs receive attention; however, the physical, emotional, spiritual, and often sexual needs are split off, causing a rift between logos and eros to expand. Being treated as an object and then, in turn, learning to treat themselves as objects in order to survive medical school leaves them wanting. Clearly, this dismissal of needs only serves to till a psychological soil with the potential for crisis to occur.

Needs are ongoing throughout our lives. When these needs are not met, the false self is developed. In my session with East, an OB-Gyn physician, the following dialogue occurred:

East stated, "Sometimes the loneliness is unbearable, and we walk into a room and our feelings are there. We have to send them away."

I asked, "Where do you send them?"

"Down and out" he replied.

"Out?" I inquired.

"Yes, out of awareness and even then, if I walk in and am in a hurtful place, they (patients) pick up on it. They don't like it; they may even tell me I don't care about them. I am not listening to them or they may leave. Next week, I will get a request for their records. I can't feel this stuff and be able to be a doctor."

I asked, "So does being a doctor mean you don't feel?"

"No" he stated, "It means I have to push the feelings away and get back to my rational mind, that is all I know to do. And then I go on to the next patient and do the same thing all over again. When you finish the day, you are whipped. There is no energy left, not for me, my wife, or my kids."

I reflected, "You are telling me you are depressing your feelings in order to get through the day, leaving you with an underlying quiet depression, possibly?" (Personal Communication, October 2016).

When depression hits, it is only a matter of time until one can no longer live in such a state. Hopefully, an opening comes, and one is able to begin the search for the divine or true self within. The potential within a person is as real today as it was the day he or she was born. The secret is to find one's way back to what was originally lost or undeveloped. Our physicians, our healers, deserve to honor their needs without shame. It is indeed our task as therapists to heighten their awareness of their own feelings, needs, and values, and with the appalling suicide rate for physicians, addressing this issue is beyond overdue.

For the physician, living in the one-sidedness of medicine has been costly. I have been fortunate enough to witness and hold space in the form of a temenos with these men and women. In this space, they find those parts of themselves that had been sent away in the service of surviving our current

medical training system where eros was deemed a weakness and un-
necessary. Their experiences are about what happens when one gives up a
part of oneself in order to survive. My observation is that their work has
been fruitful as I witnessed exiled parts of their personalities find their way
back to their feeling function, both personally and professionally. They have
come to understand that psychological suffering has come by ignoring their
deepest needs. Most importantly, they have embraced Jung's premise that
"emotion is the chief source of all becoming conscious" (Jung, 1954, p. 96,
para. 179). They became conscious by leaning into their needs.

References

Center, C. Davis, M., Detre T., Ford, D. E., Hansbrough, W., Hendin, H., &
Silverman, M. (2003). Confronting depression and suicide in physicians: A consensus statement. *Journal of the American Medical Association, 289*(23),
3161–3166. 10.1001/jama.289.23.3161.

Hillman, J. (1996). *The soul's code: In search of character and calling*. New York, NY:
Ballantine Books.

Jung, C.G. (1954). Analytical psychology and education: Three lectures. In H. Read,
M. Fordham, G. Adler, & W. McGuire (Eds.), *The collected works of C. G. Jung:
Vol. 17. The development of personality*. R.F.C. Hull (Trans.). Princeton, NJ:
Princeton University Press.

Jung, C.G. (1963). *Memories, dreams, reflections*. Aniela Jaffé (Ed.). R. Winston &
C. Winston (Trans.). New York, NY: Random House.

Jung, C.G. (1968). The psychology of the child archetype. In H. Read, M. Fordham,
G. Adler, & W. McGuire (Eds.), *The collected works of C. G. Jung: Vol. 9i. The
archetypes and the collective unconscious*. R.F.C. Hull (Trans.). Princeton, NJ:
Princeton University Press.

Jung, C.G. (1969). The soul and death. In H. Read, M. Fordham, G. Adler, & W.
McGuire (Eds.), *The collected works of C.G. Jung: Vol. 8. The structure and dynamics of the psyche*. Princeton, NJ: Princeton University Press.

Jung, C.G. (1982). *Aspects of the feminine*. Princeton, NJ: Princeton University Press.

Owens, L. (2015). *Jung in love: The mysterium in liber novus* (Monograph Edition).
Los Angeles & Salt Lake City: Gnosis Archive Books. (Originally published in:
Das Rote Buch – C.G. Juns Reise zum Andersen Pol der Welt. Thomas Arzt (Ed.).
Verlag Königshausen & Neumann, 2015).

Woodman, M. (1969). *The Stillness shall be the dancing: feminine and masculine in
emerging balance* [mp3 audio file]. College Station: Texas A & M Press. Available
electronically from http://hdl.handle.net/1969.1/86076

Chapter 7

The problem of eros and logos in medicine

I can't feel all of these feelings and still be a doctor, I have to push them down.

Physician, Personal Communication, December 1, 2016

Jung was a scientist and an empiricist, with his science encircling his most subjective task: The observation of the psyche, a direct investigation and intimate observation into his own soul as a purely "experiential process" (Jung, 1969, p. 217, para. 421). In 1913, Jung denounced his prior psychological conceptual framework as a "dead system" (Owens, 2015, p. 4). According to historian and physician Lance Owens, one of Jung's differences with Freud was regarding the concept of transference. Freud's position was that the material projected upon the doctor by the patient would invariably replicate some familial bond, typically one with mother or father. Jung saw transference as "neither a necessary nor inevitable component in every analytical relationship" (p. 17), and posited that the transference phenomena could be encountered in human affiliations outside of the patient–physician relationship. Jung thought that "Sometimes the transference evoked symbolic images rooted in deeper substrata of the unconscious, actualities that did not originate from repression of earlier life experience. These primal symbolic contents, or 'archetypes,' were natural constituents of human nature akin to instincts" (p. 17).

The hunger of the soul

As Owens related in his book *Jung in Love: The Mysterium in Liber Novus*, Jung recorded in his "Black Journals" that his most important observation in his science was the direct encounter with his own Soul; therefore, he had to be open to "direct dialogue with its mystery, itself in itself" (2015, p. 4). This mystery, said Owens, "was obtruding into his consciousness, swirling around his dreams, and causing dire visions. Jung had to meet his Soul whatever soul might be, and wherever she might lead him" (p. 4). In a journal entry dated November 12, 1913, Jung wrote,

DOI: 10.4324/9781003144502-7

> My soul, my soul, where are you? Do you hear me? I speak, I call you—
> are you there? I have returned, I am here again. I have shaken the dust
> of all the lands from my feet and I have come to you. I am with you.
> After long years of long wandering, I have come to you again. (Jung,
> 2009, p. 232)

Two nights later, he again addressed his soul:

> Who are you, child? My dreams have represented you as a child and as a
> maiden. And I found you again only through the soul of the woman. I
> am ignorant of your mystery. Look, I bear a wound that is yet not
> healed: my ambition to make an impression. Forgive me if I speak as in
> a dream, like a drunkard—are you God? (2009, p. 233 n. 49)

Owens reiterated Jung's declaration: "And I found you again only through
the soul of the woman," and said that Jung's "first hermeneutic challenge…
was bringing his experiences of the soul into the sensuous form of word and
image…. And love was a bridge to this realm. In love, Jung found a mirror
of his soul," the mirror image of the feminine (Owens, 2015, p. 5).

The two opposing elements within Jung, thinking and his unmet desire to
understand love, are reflected in the last chapter of the book *Memories,
Dreams, Reflections,* recorded and edited by Aniela Jaffé, where Jaffé recorded Jung's thoughts "regarding Eros, the god so difficult to grasp":

> In classical times, when such things were properly understood, Eros was
> considered a god whose divinity transcended our human limits, and who
> therefore could neither be comprehended nor represented in any way. I
> might, as many before me have attempted to do, venture an approach to
> this daemon, whose range of activity extends from the endless spaces of
> the heavens to the dark abysses of hell; but I falter before the task of
> finding the language which might adequately express the incalculable
> paradoxes of love. Eros is a kosmogonos, a creator and father-mother of
> all higher consciousness. I sometimes feel that Paul's words—"Though I
> speak with the tongues of men and of angels and have not love"—might
> well be the first condition of all cognition and the quintessence of divinity
> itself. Whatever the learned interpretation may be of the sentence, "God
> is love," the words affirm the complexio oppositorum of the Godhead. In
> my medical experience as well as in my own life I have again and again
> been faced with the mystery of love and have never been able to explain
> what it is. (Jung, 1963, 353)

Just as eros created a struggle in Jung's life, the absence of eros has created a
crisis for physicians. What has happened? What has gone into exile? Why
are many physicians abusing substances, having affairs, and suffering from

profound depression and anxiety? Why are they jumping off buildings and killing themselves? What has happened to those physicians who recognized the call to become a doctor at a tender age when most receptive for the seed to be planted? As innocents, they responded to the path of helping others by becoming healers without knowing what that would mean in reality. Often, the seed is related to one having a certain typology, but the climate in a family system can also be a factor, as the family is where natural wounding occurs. Common to all humanity is the introjection of family projections that form an individual's blueprint for future development. The seed for producing a scarcity of eros can sprout in such familial soil, with compensatory behaviors coming to the fore as one learns to give what one did not receive in one's formative years. The absence of eros in their families of origin again meets the budding medical student at the door of medical school, where eros is seemingly forbidden. Instead, students enter a grueling training environment that is often shaming and punitive. Not knowing what to do with any feelings other than desperately to push them down so as not to appear weak, they eventually experience a crisis of one sort or another and come to feel a lack that they do not understand. This is indicative of an undeveloped feeling function, which is the absence of the feminine, or eros. So it is that the brightest of the bright come up against something they cannot figure out. The following accounts reflect medicine's unconscious complicity in the quelling of eros.

The dissolution of medicine

A 45-year-old director of an emergency center told of his journey through the Marine Corps and graduate school, where he earned an MBA, followed by medical school. He sat in my office and confessed he did not know what to do, adding that for the first time in his life, he did not know if he wanted to be a physician any longer. He had spent ten years training to be a physician and had accumulated huge debt in the process. This career had been his dream, yet here he was, six years into his work as a physician, profoundly discouraged and questioning his choice.

When I asked him what had changed, he responded:

> Well, they don't teach you how it is going to be. They don't tell you that you will become a market commodity. You see a patient and do your best, giving them all you have, and they get to evaluate you. You get a check if the patient likes you, but if they don't, they can judge you publicly on the internet. It can even lead to being fired. It's crazy!

> I remember one night in the emergency room. I had just finished giving mouth-to-mouth to a 17-year-old. I couldn't bring him back. He died. When I went to the next patient room, the man cussed me out and spit on

me because he had to wait to be treated for a sinus infection. I didn't become a physician to get spit on, then evaluated like a commodity that can be bought and used in the marketplace. It's sad that my calling to be a physician now seems more like prostitution.

The only thing that keeps me going now is the great relationships I have with my staff. Yet when I hear techs say they want to go to medical school, I want to say to them get your education, but do something else. The nurses are like me, too—burned out and unhappy. I can't believe I'm saying all of this to you. But this is the truth. I hate where I am in life right now. I am so disappointed in medicine. And the saddest part is all of my physician friends feel the same way I do. (Personal Communication, February 15, 2016)

In his study of modern medicine and the healing process, Rosen (2003) identified loneliness as one of the effects of practicing medicine and concluded that without meaningful interaction, loss of eros is experienced. Often, physicians come into my office reporting an agonizing loneliness and despair, much like the emergency room physician in the story above. It is my contention that this loneliness reflects a deep yearning for a part of themselves they are missing or have lost. This yearning is unconscious in that it reflects an undeveloped, foreign aspect of themselves and grief over a separation that cannot be repaired by simply adding the pieces back together. As historian of religion Mircea Eliade (1976) wrote, "life cannot be repaired, it can only be re-created by a return to sources." Again, I refer to Jung's postulation that loneliness is the inability to communicate the things that seem important to oneself or results from risking standing alone in a certain point of view.

The training of physicians is almost exclusively focused on utilization of the thinking function at the expense of an inner life. This singular focus creates an opening for psychological crises to occur; however, the successful negotiation of crises can foster psychological growth in the physician leading to a greater capacity to relate. Growth in the service of the feeling function creates a space for nurturance, compassion, insight, intuition, wisdom, and the capacity to heal. Without growth, in a Depth Psychological sense, the lack of eros leaves physicians wanting for what they do not know, which is the holding feminine principle.

Carl Jung saw the movement of eros moving both individuals to a new realm... Eros always works toward new ground in both, unknown, unfamiliar, and always having to do with the future. Lockhart, in his book *Words as Eggs* (1983), supports this through a quote from Jung in a letter written on April 18, 1941: "Eros becomes not transference, not ordinary friendship or sympathy, but more primitive, more primeval, more spiritual than anything we can describe. It is immediate presence, as if we were mixed together in some way" (Jung, 1973, p. 298).

Jung directed attention to the dark side of eros when he stated, "Logically, the opposite of love is hate, and or eros, Phobos (fear); but psychologically it is the will to power" (1953, p. 53, para. 78). Some years later, he wrote, "An unconscious eros always expresses itself as will to power" (1959, p. 88, para. 167). He saw the opposite of eros to be the masculine aspect of the personality that is aligned with logos. Logos is logic, which is related to words being put into syntax to express thoughts and is also linear. Jung addresses the relationship of eros and logos in *The Philosophical Tree* (1968a) as one needs the other. Without understanding, love alone is useless. They balance each other. Logos compensates for eros with differentiation, clarification, discrimination, and detachment while eros weaves and conveys an relatedness.

Jungian analyst and Episcopalian priest J. Pittman McGehee, in his book, *The Paradox of Love* (2011), concurred with this idea as he posited that eros creates logos and brings it into consciousness by bringing the masculine and feminine together. We have the rational side of the medical model, which can better facilitate healing with the integration of the feminine.

In her 2016 lecture, "Interest and Boredom," Verena Kast described this exchange by suggesting the following continuum. At one end is the self, and at the opposite end is the other, with the ego-complex placed in the middle, which looks something like this:

Self_____Ego complex_____Other

Within the self is the spark or carrier charged with individual destiny, which lies within the physician, as it does all of us. While this spark exists, one is not free to choose one's own destiny; however, it is one's consciousness that makes one free to accept it. As Jung taught, we do not choose what happens to us, but we can choose how we want to respond to what happens to us. This is to say we are in fact co-creators, not of our fate but certainly of our destiny. In the psychology of the physician, imagine, in the diagram above, the "self" as holding the calling of the physician and the "other" as representing the patient. The middle, representing the ego complex, represents activities, always moving and changing, which is the leading emotion for the physician in the development of creativity. Swiss psychiatrist and Jungian expert, Dr. Alfred Ribi might suggest the use of the sensate function as the first engagement of the self with the other, followed by accessing the thinking or feeling function. Then the thinking and feeling functions can be employed through the working of the ego.

It is significant to note the difficulty of this process for the physician who is entering patient data in the presence of the patient and is aware of being bound by the "15 minutes per patient" protocol, when only seven minutes are left. Also, during this constricted time period, the physician may be worrying if his or her diagnosis is sufficient for the patient to get insurance reimbursement as well as worrying about meeting a quota of 65 patients seen per day? This unrelenting pressure and stress are evident in the following story a cardiologist shared with me:

> *The hospital administrators are checking my numbers every day. Yesterday, I saw 63 patients. Care is no longer the focus—money is. I signed a five-year contract with the hospital, and if I don't meet their quotas, I lose my admitting privileges. I hate it and feel trapped.*
>
> *On top of this burden, hospital politics come into play. When I tried to surrender my contract, the hospital immediately began to put pressure on my wife, who is also a physician. How did they put pressure on her? She was supposed to have a rotating medical student in the operating room just to observe, and they blocked her, even though she had all the necessary paperwork. She had had this arrangement for some years and suddenly it was curtailed, not because of her, as she had not signed a contract with the hospital. Her operating room activities were blocked because of me. What is sad is this goes on with other physicians. Everyday. Everywhere.*
>
> *Until I started working with you [in my therapy with him], I didn't know what I was feeling. I managed my anxiety by fixing a drink as soon as I got home, followed by wine with dinner, then a couple of nightcaps afterward. Now I know it is anxiety, and under that anxiety is a ton of anger. One of the ways this manifested was by treating my patients in a disagreeable way. I felt distraught upon realizing this and now understand how difficult it is to be that kind of physician. I don't want to be in a system that focuses on the production of patient numbers. Patients are lined up every day like it's a factory, and I want to treat them like men and women, and that's a challenge. It's just dehumanizing for the physician and the patient.*
> (Personal Communication, December 2017)

This physician's calling has become a burden, and it is difficult under this type of pressure to develop a relationship with a patient. Eros is clearly absent while logos dominates, precluding any sense of satisfaction and self-worth. Under the current medical model, it is clear that the eros has been lost in the service of money going to the insurance companies, to the corporate hospitals, and sometimes to the physicians themselves. The ethics chairman of a local hospital recently reported that the hospital was receiving complaints from the patients and their families as the young hospital staff were inept and ill prepared when explaining a terminal condition to patients.

The psychology of transference

To regain equilibrium between logos and eros, learning to navigate the workings of the psyche is critical. As previously stressed, we need each other

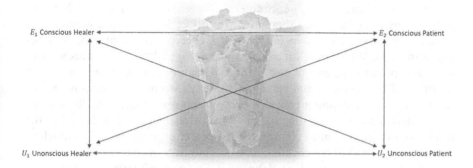

Figure 7.1 Energy and the unconscious.

in relationship. In considering relationship, Jung's model of transference addresses the multilayered process that holds the potential for a shift in today's medical culture. It is worth noting again Jung' proposition that "the meeting of two personalities is like the contact of two chemical substances: if there is any reaction, both are transformed. We cannot change anything until we accept it" (1933, p. 49). The model shown in Figure 7.1 reveals what the unconscious has to offer, whereby the necessary eros might find its way into the healing dyad (Jung, 1985b).

In this model, E(1) refers to the ego of the physician, or the physician's conscious sense of him- or herself; E(2) refers to the ego of the patient, or the patient's conscious sense of him- or herself; and U(1) and U(2) are the psychological histories of the physician and the patient, respectively, including what has happened to them since birth, especially in the field of relationship, most of which is unconscious.

This diagram indicates that there are 12 directions in which the energy may travel, only two of which are conscious, with two more that may become conscious. The energy can flow from E(1) to E(2) (ego to ego) in either direction. It may also flow in either direction from E(1) to U(1) and E(2) to U(2). Furthermore, when the U (unconscious) of either party is engaged—and it always is to a greater or lesser degree—its contents will be projected onto the E (conscious) of the other, represented here by the two diagonal lines.

The diagram (Figure 7.1) reveals that the encounter occurs when the patient and physician meet. The patient enters the encounter with a need and projects the archetype of the healer onto the physician, often in an unconscious, somewhat childish manner. In response, the physician may project the child archetype onto the patient. In these archetypal situations, an individual perceives and acts according to a basic paradigm inherent in him- or herself but also present in all humanity. Guggenbühl-Craig (2015) discussed how these projections represent a common problem: Patients have an unrealistic view of the physician, and Jung encourages the professional to accept projection as a natural facet of interpersonal encounters. Guggenbühl-Craig added that projections simply appear when they must. In this exchange of transference and countertransference, the physician–patient archetype enters into the field between the two. When Jung's medical students asked him how to respond to such an experience, he encouraged them to be natural, spontaneous, open, and undefended by a professional persona. In today's world of Western medicine, this would mean creating a place for eros, which is a problem, as the current system makes no space or time for this type of relatedness. It is here that the trajectory of medicine must change, for the power of medicine has as much to do with psychological insight (feminine energy) as scientific knowledge.

In the construct above, Jung delineated a process whereby conscious and unconscious material flows. How might this look in the patient–physician dyad? I am imagining a male–female dyad to demonstrate the physicians' fear of this flow. If the physician is male and the patient is female, a complex of feeling-toned energy is often experienced by both. That is to say, a female patient is attracted to the animus of the male physician. The animus, of course, can be either positive or negative, but for the purposes of this book, I am supposing that the female patient experiences the male physician as a positive animus, meaning a positive projection of the female's unconscious animus onto the physician. At the same time, what may be happening within the psyche of the male physician is the igniting of the anima, which, for the purposes of this book, is also considered as a positive projection. When this type of projection occurs between the physician and the patient, positive energy is exchanged. When asked what to do with this energy, Jung proposed being aware of it so that it might be brought into the relationship, if necessary (Jung, 1985a).

When the unconscious histories of the physician and patient are activated, the dynamics of transference and countertransference are evoked in a particular way. Either one could feel a strong dis-ease or, alternatively, a strong attraction. When this energy is brought to consciousness, it opens up an opportunity for psychological growth, making room for an inner type of healing regardless of the reduction of the symptoms or a cure. A story recently told to me reflects this teaching.

An oncological surgeon and his young resident were making rounds on a 70-year-old patient on whom they had operated the previous day. As they were speaking with her, the original gynecologist entered the patient's room, and thus, all three physicians were in her presence when she addressed the original gynecologist. She called him by name and said, "I hear what you are telling me but your body language tells me something else," to which he responded, "Mrs. Johnson," as he touched her hand, "you have been my patient for seven years. I know you, I know your husband, I know your children. And when something is going on with you, it is going on with me."

This was a physician who clearly heard his patient, felt the conscious and unconscious activation, and chose to bring the care to consciousness. Regarding projection, Jung declared, "The general psychological reason for projection is always an activated unconscious that seeks expression" (1976, p. 152, para. 352). Often, I am asked by physicians why this occurs. I answer by again referencing the wisdom of Jung:

> Strictly speaking, projection is never made: it happens, it is simply there. In the darkness of anything external to me I find, without recognizing it as such, an interior or psychic life that is my own... Such projections repeat themselves whenever man tries to explore an empty darkness and involuntarily fills it with living form. (1968b, p. 245, para. 346)

Over the years, I have learned from physicians that they feel overly responsible for the patient, at the expense of getting their own needs met. It is essential that physicians come to recognize this. In order for eros to be in balance with logos, a physician needs to understand what is going on in his or her own psyche, as indicated in the above example—this is to say, understanding what they are feeling so that they may allow their feeling function or eros to guide them. I emphatically inform physicians of the necessity to bring eros into their relationship with patients, and that through psychological awareness, they can be taught to hold the energy of eros within a temenos in an appropriately vulnerable way during their exchange with patients. One can only do this kind of work if one is confident in oneself, which simply means to be always in the process of doing one's own inner work. In the end, it is through eros that one determines what one sees in the other. For physicians, this energy of eros connects them to the divine spark that held the original call to become a physician. The more a physician is in touch with his or her feeling function, the more he or she can be present to his patient. It is not necessary that the physician be all knowing, working out of logos exclusively; rather, it is important for a physician to be connected to all four functions: Sensate, intuition, feeling, and thinking. Only then can the gold of relationship come forth. Through eros, physicians can learn to access empathy for their patients, their colleagues, and themselves.

Throughout my years of experience in working with physicians, I have observed first-hand the ways in which the tenets of analytical psychology have profoundly enhanced the lives of these bright men and women who entered medicine to be healers. In this transformative process, they have come to know eros as necessary for meeting the needs of the other as well as themselves. Jungian psychology holds that when two people meet, it is the totality of their psyches that enter the space between them: Conscious and unconscious, spoken and unspoken. All these desires, fantasies, feelings, and emotions enter into play but are rarely stated or directly expressed. Because the tension created by these factors is present in every interaction between the physician and patient, it is imperative that the currently one-sided practice of Western medicine achieve an integration of logos and eros in a meaningful and transformative way.

References

Eliade, M. (1976). *A history of religious ideas: Vol. 1. From the stone age to the Eleusinian mysteries*. W.R. Trask (Trans.). Chicago, IL: University of Chicago Press.

Guggenbühl-Craig, A. (2015). *Power in the helping professions*. M. Gubitz (Trans.). Dallas, TX: Spring.

Jung, C.G. (1933). *Modern man in search of a soul*. Orlando, FL: Houghton Mifflin Harcourt Publishing Company.

Jung, C.G. (1953). On the Psychology of the Unconscious. In H. Read, M. Fordham, G. Adler, & W. McGuire (Eds.), *The collected works of C. G. Jung: Vol. 7. Two essays in analytical psychology*. R.F.C. Hull (Trans.). Princeton, NJ: Princeton University Press.

Jung, C.G. (1959). Psychological aspects of the mother archetype. In H. Read, M. Fordham, G. Adler, & W. McGuire (Eds.), *The collected works of C.G. Jung: Vol. 9i. The archetypes and the collective unconscious*. R.F.C. Hull (Trans.). Princeton, NJ: Princeton University Press.

Jung, C.G. (1963). *Memories, dreams, reflections*. Aniela Jaffé (Ed.). R. Winston & C. Winston (Trans.). New York, NY: Random House.

Jung, C.G. (1968a). The philosophical tree. (R.F.C. Hull, Trans.). In H. Read, M. Fordham, G. Adler, & W. McGuire (Eds.), *The collected works of C. G. Jung: Vol. 13. Alchemical studies*. R.F.C. Hull (Trans.). Princeton, NJ: Princeton University Press.

Jung, C.G. (1968b). Religious ideas in alchemy. In H. Read, M. Fordham, G. Adler, & W. McGuire (Eds.), *The collected works of C. G. Jung: Vol. 12. Psychology and alchemy*. R.F.C. Hull (Trans.). Princeton, NJ: Princeton University Press.

Jung, C.G. (1969). On the nature of the psyche. In H. Read, M. Fordham, G. Adler, & W. McGuire (Eds.), *The collected works of C.G. Jung: Vol. 8. The structure and dynamics of the psyche*. R.F.C. Hull (Trans.). Princeton, NJ: Princeton University Press.

Jung, C.G. (1973).*Letters, vol. 1: 1906–1950*. G. Adler, A. Jaffé, & R.F.C. Hull (Trans.). Princeton, NJ: Princeton University Press.

Jung, C.G. (1976). The Tavistock lectures. In H. Read, M. Fordham, G. Adler, & W. McGuire (Eds.), *The collected works of C.G. Jung: Vol. 18. The symbolic life*. R.F.C. Hull (Trans.). Princeton, NJ: Princeton University Press.

Jung, C.G. (1985a). *The collected works of C.G. Jung: Vol. 6. Psychological types*. H. Read, M. Fordham, G. Adler, & W. McGuire (Eds.). R.F.C. Hull (Trans.). Princeton, NJ: Princeton University Press.

Jung, C.G. (1985b). The psychology of the transference. In H. Read, M. Fordham, G. Adler, & W. McGuire (Eds.), *The collected works of C.G. Jung: Vol. 16. The practice of psychotherapy*. R.F.C. Hull (Trans.). Princeton, NJ: Princeton University Press.

Jung, C.G. (2009). *The red book: Liber novus*. S. Shamdasani, (Ed). S. Shamdasani, J. Peck, M. Kyburz (Trans.). New York, NY: W.W. Norton & Co.

Kast, V. (2016). Interest and boredom. Lecture at the C.G. Jung Institute. Kusnacht, Switzweland.

Lockhart, R.A. (1983). *Words as eggs*. Dallas, TX: Spring Publications.

McGehee, J.P. (2011). *The paradox of love: A Jungian look at the dynamics of life's greatest mystery*. Houston, TX: Bright Sky Press.

Owens, L. (2015). *Jung in love: The mysterium in liber novus* (Monograph Edition). Los Angeles, CA & Salt Lake City, UT: Gnosis Archive Books. (Originally published in: *Das Rote Buch – C.G. Juns Reise zum Andersen Pol der Welt*. T. Arzt (Ed.). Verlag Königshausen & Neumann, 2015).

Rosen, D.H. (2003, November 22). Modern medicine and the healing process. *The Jung Page*. Retrieved from: http://www.cgjungpage.org/learn/articles/analytical-psychology/101-modern-medicine-and-the-healing-process

Chapter 8

The shadow side of medicine

> *The doctor can only work creatively if he bears in mind that despite all his knowledge and technique, in the final analysis, he must always strive to constellate the healing factor in the patient.*
> Adolf Guggenbühl-Craig, Power in the Helping Professions

According to Jung, the shadow contains things one does not know or does not like about oneself as well as positive possibilities within that are unknown. Once when teaching a seminar at the Jung Institute in Zurich, Jung encouraged his students to be open, natural, undefended by the professional persona. He taught that in the helping professions, the shadow will always be present in the relationship and encouraged the students to become aware of the shadow material and admit the shadow into the interpersonal field. Both the positive and negative sides of the shadow are apparent in the following narrative from my consultation with an oncological surgeon regarding a difficult situation with a patient. This account illustrates what can occur when a physician leans into consciousness in the face of the collective shadow of medicine. Here is the story the physician Jonas told me, followed by our interaction:

I have a 70-year-old patient, a nurse by profession, who has been my patient for ten years. At the end of a recent appointment, she asked for my opinion about an outside matter. She related having had a surgical procedure elsewhere, after which she developed an infection. She met with the physician in question to discuss the infection, and he indicated the infection was nothing to worry about. Later, she called that same physician three times, and he did not return her call. Eventually, another physician from the same practice called her, and she expressed her concern regarding her infection, how this might have happened, as well as the lack of responsiveness by her surgeon. She was not well received and not satisfied with his response. Not feeling heard, she contacted the administrator at the hospital where the surgery had been performed and again was not satisfied with the

DOI: 10.4324/9781003144502-8

response. She then contacted a lawyer who told her she did not have a case. She then contacted the state medical board to lodge a formal complaint about her experience with the operating physician.

On my end, I felt like she was looking for ammunition for a lawsuit, which I had no interest in. This irritated me, as I had known this surgeon for many years and knew him to be extremely competent. When I shared my opinion of him, she got mad at me. I explained that I had gotten an infection after a surgery on my finger and stated that these things happen. Two days later, I got a letter from her that stated I had let her down, and then she reminded me that I had been her doctor for ten years, and she never thought she would see this side of me. She told me that I was like all the others and said, "You doctors all stick together," adding that I had refused to respond to her, like all of the other doctors. I called the surgeon in question, relating the events of her office visit with me and the letter she wrote afterward, and he told me, "Just fire her from your practice. That's what we did. You can never make this woman happy. At the very least, don't respond to her. Ignore her."

I called several other colleagues, and they said the same thing. They said there were plenty of patients and to just get rid of her. This bothered me, and I don't know what to do about it. (Personal Communication, February 2018)

As our session continued, Jonas processed his dislike of confrontations and his distress at not knowing how to respond to this patient. From our previous discussions, he understood that his feelings were there to help him know what he values. His response was that he valued this patient, but he had no idea how to respond to the scathing letter. Then he asked me to teach him another way, as he did not want to "fire" or ignore her.

The maturity of grace

I reflected for a moment and thought: A master physician is one who is in touch with his feelings. At the age of 73, Jonas was mature yet still open to learning how to care for his patients without identifying with the God-like projection many place onto physicians. I knew him to be a man of compassion and humility, with a willingness to enter into the territory of conflict and relationship. This physician found a way to be vulnerable to his patient's emotional pain even though this elicited discomfort in him.

Jonas finally decided that a telephone call to the woman was appropriate, in which the message was "You matter" and "How are you doing?" In turn, she responded by apologizing for her behavior as well as the letter she had written him and then told him he was a good doctor. Jonas found the courage to step away from the collective shadow of the medical model, which, in this case, involved the disregard and "firing" of a patient by the other physicians in the service of convenience. At the same time, Jonas came to know an aspect of his shadow in a positive sense, as he faced his dislike for confrontation.

Furthermore, Jonas had held the tension of the opposites found in the other physicians' advice juxtapositioned against his feelings for his patient. In doing so, he caught a glimpse of the transcendent function by finding a third thing, or way, in the resolution of the conflict. It is curious that the physicians who fired the patient unconsciously seemed to imply that one could only be their patient if one did not get mad at them. In the world of medicine, acting in a narcissistic way toward a patient is part of the collective shadow. How effective is a surgeon if he or she uses only one hand? I suggest that what this woman experienced was "one-handed" medicine, whereby the physicians in question only thought to dismiss her from their practice. Jonas was able to connect eros and logos when he expressed, "You must feel very, very alone." In this simple act, he joined her.

Once, I accompanied a friend with terminal cancer to an appointment with her oncologist. Stacy, who had Stage IV cancer, had raved not only about this physician's kindness and gentle care but also his advocacy for her when dealing with insurance companies. She knew I was researching the world of physicians and wanted me to meet him. When we entered his office, he greeted her with a loving hug and was clearly glad to see her. He asked how her family was as well as how she was adjusting to retirement. Moving to the topic of her treatment, Stacy said she wanted to tell him a dream she had, to which he nodded assent. Stacy then shared a dream from two weeks prior:

> I was at the Crescent Moon Retreat Center on the floor creating a great tapestry of art. There was a knock at the front door of the lodge. Someone opened the door and two police officers walked in. One was carrying a garment bag. I knew there was a long and flowing dress inside the bag and that it was for me. I asked, "Why have you come?" and one of the officers said, "We have come for you, Stacy. It's time for you to go with us." I got up, leaving my creative project on the floor, and left the lodge with them.
> (Personal Communication, February 2016)

With her understanding of Jungian psychology, Stacy knew how to work with her dreams, and she suspected this dream was a "death dream." From a Jungian perspective, when one dreams of taking off or putting on new clothes or leaving old clothes, the dream is often speaking of transition from this life to the next. For Stacy, the police officers knocking at the door meant that her transition would be safe and that she had no need to be afraid. What had begun as her creative project here in this life was now ending as she left the lodge under the protection of the police officers.

Silence fell over the exam room after she spoke her dream, and I saw a single tear rolling down her oncologist's cheek. I looked down when I noticed his lower lip slightly quivering. She said, "I want to stop taking the trial medications. I'm losing feeling in my feet, and I don't want to spend my last months of life in a wheelchair." She spoke with an unbelievably firm grace. As she did so, the oncologist pulled his stool to be even with her on the examining table. He took her hands and restated what she had just said to him and then, in a gentle voice, explained what she could expect without the trial medications. Again, there was a profound silence, and I then saw a tear fall down Stacy's cheek. Quietly, she told him she wanted to live fully until she died. He never took his eyes away from hers. At that moment, I knew I was in the presence of a holy moment. The beauty in the room was so illuminating and full that I could barely breathe as I sat in quiet witness. It was as if my eyes were too human to behold this depth of love. I sat with my head down until I heard my dear friend say, "And now that that is settled, I want you to help Suzanne know what it's like to be a physician. I want her to know you. We need more physicians like you in the world." He looked over at me and nodded in agreement. I quietly said, "Thank you." I cannot think of a more numinous description of the positive shadow in a physician, relinquishing his control over the patient as she took into control her own process of death. This physician was able to access the possibility of being present with his patient and being a witness to her process without exerting his control. This story expresses how transformative it is to integrate positive aspects of self when they are brought to consciousness through suffering, and it reflects Jung's idea as rendered by Jungian analyst Lawrence Staples (2008): "The shadow, where we hide our sins in secret, is 90 percent gold."

Unlike the story told above, the following is a physician's account of the reticence he experienced when called upon to be honest and direct and his painful journey in learning how to tell patients they were going to die:

> *I was about to learn the impact of what we were not taught in medical school. A single mother of three children presented in my office complaining of back pain. Only, 47 years old, she had a previous diagnosis of breast cancer. Given her history and the severity of her pain, I ordered a full body scan which revealed her bones were riddled with metastatic disease. I told her I would call her with the results the next day as I didn't want to tell her her prognosis. Knowing I would be out of town the next day, I left the task for my covering partner to convey the results. My partner, thinking I had already told her the results, did not address her in person, but had left a new prescription with the nurse. It was then, after she returned home and researched the new medicine that she realized that this medicine was prescribed for terminal cancer.*(Personal Communication, March 2015)

This story illustrates another aspect of shadow in the medical school system. Why are physicians not taught the sensitive process involved in telling patients, in a soulful way, that they are going to die? When communication contains the element of relatedness or eros, a sacred space or temenos is created between two people. This space holds more than just the words being expressed, for words are sometimes limited. It also creates an opportunity for our most basic human needs to be seen and heard, illuminating the value of both people involved in the process. When unable to speak about what is happening between two people, we create loneliness and a breakdown of intimacy. How can this vacuum hidden in the shadow of medical school training be remedied? How can physicians be taught to see the woundedness of their patients in themselves? As Jung has taught us, only the wounded healer heals. An obstetrician-gynecologist makes the following observations about relatedness:

> *We are not taught how to do this in medical school. We are actually taught not to have a relationship with our patients. We want to do this, but we are afraid of how much time it will take, but I have watched you [addressing me] do this, and it really takes less time when you make that connection. We have been taught to send the emotion away. I want you to continue to bring this to our practice for our physicians. Your work has also given me permission to deal with surgical complications in a way that is helpful to me. And you have taught us how to deal with our fellow physician more effectively. Lonely? I am one of 3,000 physicians who are mothers [in an online community]. My support system is the internet. Until you started working with us, we thought we were the only ones working this hard, but then we came to realize that no one gets by without being human and all the feelings associated with that. We have been taught to "suck it up," when we need the help. This leaves us no place to turn. My connection with fellow female physicians who are mothers has been a godsend.* (Personal Communication, 2012)

The fear of judgment and public reproach relegates these physicians into a common exile. They have found community and validation in their experience as mothers and physicians that balance care of their patients with the care of their family as they support each other online.

After 25 years as a physician, Rachel Remen has also discovered it is possible to be a professional and still live from the heart. Again, it is not something she learned in medical school, as she related to me while attending a workshop in 2009.

> *We were taught that the expression of emotions is viewed as clouding a physician's judgment, which contributes to incompetent care. No matter what we do, finding fulfillment may require cultivating the capacity of the heart in the same way we pursue new knowledge. We still need to connect intimately to the life around us. Knowledge alone will not help us live well. We need to take off "the mask" to do that.* (Personal Communication, 2016)

Although medical training instills scientific objectivity and distance, other perspectives are considered suspect or even dangerous. Over time, Remen has come to believe that being human with emotions connects physicians to patients more effectively.

Remen clearly understands the concept of persona and its professional necessity; however, she also understands that this "mask" can cover part of the humanity of the individual behind it. Medical schools need to teach the importance of balancing scientific knowledge with the depth of the soul so that physicians can learn how to be truly present to one another in a meaningful way.

According to Dr. Alfred Ribi,

> Medical doctors are sensitive and need to be accepted as they are. They need to understand that it is normal to have problems as problems belong to life. The attitude toward the problem can be difficult. This is where the persona comes in. The medical school professor may present himself as having no problems and teaches the medical student that he or she should not have problems as well. This is only persona—not real personality. Everyone has problems, and it is not a bad thing to have problems. (Personal Communication, 2009)

Identifying boundaries

Another difficult topic for physicians is negotiating boundaries. In Jungian terms, this refers to holding the tension of the opposites, logos and eros, in clinical encounters between physician and patient. Using the language of the physician, a healthy balance might be likened to a cell membrane, which involves an active process, requiring energy that decides what to let in and what to let out. A cell membrane is semipermeable and does not keep everything inside of it or keep everything out. In terms of physicians' boundaries, negotiating this balance requires continual decision-making, and learning this process can facilitate meaningful connections with patients.

It is my contention that not only do physicians have to learn to balance their exchange with patients, they must also learn to be permeable like a cell membrane in their interactions with other physicians. By that I mean, they must learn to monitor the exchange in the service of personal integrity. The following story told to me by a surgical oncologist explains how physician-to-physician interaction can become problematic and challenge the integrity of the professional relationships:

> Dr. Jones would call and ask for help in surgery. When the surgery occurred, I would end up doing most, if not all of the work, with him sometimes assisting me. When the time for billing would roll around,

Dr. Jones would bill as the surgeon and would code me as the assistant. This happened more times than I care to recall. Finally, about ten years ago, I learned what to let in and what not to allow. I learned to say if the procedure involved a cancer, then my office has certain codes to use for billing. This lets the other physician know that I am not going to be taken advantage of. (Personal Communication 2017)

The physician who told this story reported that he routinely teaches his fellows how to manage the container between physicians. He was clear that he was not at all taught how to take care of himself in medical school. It, therefore, appears that in the medical culture, the betrayal of the self begins in an unconscious way, creating fear and dependency. This dependency occurs when a young doctor is relying upon other physicians' referrals for his or her sense of well-being. The specialty surgeon in the story above was dependent upon the referrals of other physicians. Without a clear understanding of appropriate permeability within his psyche, these relationships have the potential to become destructive.

More important is the play of parental complexes in the psyche of the physician, which can come to the surface in the medical environment. Physicians must learn the underpinnings of their complexes in order to walk the tightrope of caring for their own well-being. That is to say, when the call comes for help from a colleague, it should be not only the joining of two personalities with the common goal of caring for the patient. As a way to manage his or her anxiety, the new physician will naturally want to fuse with the more experienced physician rather than maintaining his or her own separate identity; therefore, it is important for the more experienced physician to hold the integrity of the boundary.

The shadow in the collective medical culture must be addressed. We must let go of the projection of "shining armor" onto physicians and instead teach them to embrace their vulnerability, doubt, and imperfection. The collective medical culture's obliteration of the humanity of the physician no longer serves the kingdom. In the end, we need a medical culture that views embracing the individual humanity of physicians not as an obstacle but rather a precondition for being an effective healer. It is my contention that analytical psychology holds the key.

References

Guggenbühl-Craig, A. (2009). *Power in the helping professions.* M. Gubitz (Trans.). Dallas, TX: Spring.

Staples, L. (2008). *Guilt with a twist: The Promethean way.* Sheridan, WY: Fisher King Press.

Chapter 9

The wounded sexuality of today's physician

How is it possible to get across from the sexual... to the spiritual not only from the scientific standpoint, but as a phenomenon in the individual?
C.G. Jung, Analytical Psychology: Notes of the Seminar Given in 1925

Many physicians tend to be split off from their own bodies and identify with the light of science and the intellect. This orientation puts them in danger of acting out the unconscious split between body and psyche. The truth is that they have been taught to focus on other people's bodies via their brain, leaving a hungry ghost hidden beneath their white coats. Limited life force or eros is experienced if they remain fixed in this psychological state, which precludes resolving the psyche–soma split. Once this split is consciously identified, it is imperative that the feeling function not be dismissed. Jung identified the downside of the opposites not coming together: "To attack symptoms or, as it is now called, symptom analysis... [is] only half the story, and... the real point is the treatment of the whole psychic human being" (1966, p. 89, para. 199). Healing is denied for both physician and patient if this split is not resolved. As opposites, sexuality and spirituality create a tension on each end of a continuum. Without aligning at either end, if one is able to hold this tension, a transcendent third appears as the creative gift.

Projection

The following story illustrates how one side of the physician was split when the tension could not be maintained. Once, when I was teaching about feelings and attraction to a group of physicians, I asked one of the young male physicians how he responds to a woman while medically examining her exposed attractive breasts. He replied that he did not see them as breasts and added that they were just body parts. I asked him if he really expected me to believe him, and when he answered, "Yes," I noticed his breathing became shallower and his face flushed. I thought to myself: *This physician has*

DOI: 10.4324/9781003144502-9

learned to split. He can tell himself that the beautiful breasts are just body parts, but his feeling side feels something he is too afraid to own.

I asked him if he could simply say to himself, "This is a body of beauty, these breasts are beautiful, and I can respect and acknowledge that." I explained that this seemed more humane than denying one's own experience. It is clear that physicians are in desperate need of learning how to acknowledge their feeling function and, in doing so, learn how to deal with what arises. The following dialogue occurred in a physicians' group with whom I have met weekly since 1986. Some of the participants have now retired, and new ones have joined, but the flow of the group continues to bring life to these physicians, ages 34 to 72. A female gynecological surgeon, whom I shall call Mary, opened the group dialogue.

Mary: I need to talk. I've had it. I can't stand to have sex this way one more time. This has been going on for 18 years in our bedroom. Let me correct that. 18 years ago, it would have started in the kitchen while I was trying to cook dinner. John [a pseudonym] would grab me on the butt, and I would react by telling him, "I am not a piece of meat." He would giggle and stop, only to re-engage with the same behavior later that week. While it took a while, today he doesn't grab my butt or breasts. But I'm talking about our sex life and notice I didn't say lovemaking. I'm okay if he does what he does once in a while, but not every time. I hate it! No more! (She took a deep breath and started to weep.)

Dr. Hales: Can you tell me about your tears?

Mary: He starts by rubbing my back. It always starts there. I have told him before, "Please don't expect sex when you rub my back." He doesn't rub my back to relax me, he rubs my back to arouse himself, and then after a while, he rolls me over. We never kiss, and I want to kiss him. If I try to kiss him, he places his mouth over my breast. That is okay, but I want to see his face. Then he penetrates me, but before ejaculating or I reach orgasm, he pulls out, flips me over, and ejaculates on my back. I am sick of this. I want to have frontal penetration, and I want to look at him. I love him. I want him to look at me and see that I am here. I feel left out and excluded. That's why I'm crying. It makes me feel sad, like something is wrong with me.

I allow Mary the space to feel her feelings, which seem to be about sadness and shame. After a few moments, I ask her what she is feeling.

Mary: I don't feel love, I don't feel seen—it is like I don't exist. It's awful. There is nothing more I can do to get him to see me. It's like I don't matter.

Dr. Hales: (I gently suggested she was describing the emotion of shame.) Can you take me back to a time when you were a little girl when you might have felt this sadness?

I notice her breathing has slowed down, and she is looking toward her left, which tells me she is reviewing memories.

Mary: (With a deep sob) Yes, my daddy, left and I wanted to go with him, but my mom couldn't take care of me. After he left, my stepdad molested me.

Dr. Hales: I can only imagine how deeply hurt you were being left in an unsafe place, where you were being hurt with no one there for you. No one to see you, no one to hear you—a place of almost intolerable loneliness and pain. A place of great betrayal, first by your dad who left you, then your mom who did not protect you, and then by your stepdad who molested you. A great, gaping, vast emptiness, where no one is there for you. Mary, can you go to that child, that little girl who wants her daddy to see her, can you go there in your mind's eye to that memory? In your imagination, can you see the competent adult you, the woman you are today, and walk into that memory and see that little girl begging to be chosen? Can you see her and you, the adult Mary, at the same time?

Mary: Yes.

Dr. Hales: What is it you feel when you see this child?

Mary: I want to go get her.

Dr. Hales: Call her by name, drop to your knees, and open your arms to her. Does she come to you?

Mary: Yes... She seems sad.

Dr. Hales: What does the child need?

Mary: She needs to be loved and someone needs to take her out of there. She runs to me and I embrace her.

Dr. Hales: Can you take the little girl out of this place? Can you see the child merging with you into your own heart?

Mary: (Weeps openly.)

Dr. Hales: Whatever this child needed then is what she is needing now. That is why this memory came. This child has waited a lifetime for you. She only wants you. She can no longer get this from outside of her, from someone else. This must come from you. She wants you to see her, and hear her, and be interested in her. She wants you to choose her. Are you willing to do that with her? Imagine just holding this child and telling her, I am here for you. I want you. Your needs are okay with me, and I will protect you. Tell her you will never leave her. (Personal Communication, 2018)

Mary simply nodded. Her spirit was quiet and calm as tears streamed down her face. At some level, she knew she had just chosen herself and could learn how to trust and protect herself. In this way, she would learn how to trust others in her life. After beginning with agitated energy, the group energy now shifted from fear to calming gentleness.

Mary may now be ready to understand that John may be capable of meeting some of her needs some of the time, but in those times when he cannot, she must be able to respond to the child within herself, instead of looking for someone else to choose her all of the time. This is the valuing principle of the feeling function in Jungian psychology: It simply tells us what is important to us.

Mary displays the state of being split from her body, her feelings or eros, and her own vulnerability. She only feels alive when she is making love in absolute release to another. She wants desperately to be loved but is fearful of being loved. These simultaneous conflicting needs make no sense to her conscious ego. What does this interaction between Mary and her husband have to do with sex? This issue with intimacy is often confused with sexual performance and shows up repeatedly in group as well as individual sessions with physicians and others. Why does it show up as a sexual issue? The answer is simple—it is part of the dilemma of being human. Thus, asking for wholeness of spirituality. Here, again, are the opposites. It is in all of our marriages.

Often in our Western culture, pressure is placed on sexuality and sexual performance to heal the wound of connection, relatedness, or spirituality. We have been slow to learn that we can have biological sex without our feeling function. Perhaps better said, we have known for a long time how to be sexual without feeling, but we have not known how to have sex with feelings. To be fully aware of our feelings, we must be grounded in our bodies, in a state that is called embodiment. We dissociate from our bodies when we are uncomfortable with our feelings; instead, we stay in our heads, focusing on performance. As members of this culture, we are having a great deal of sex, but we are performing it without embodiment, without being present with our feelings, without soul. To be embodied requires honoring the feeling function. Physicians are taught to honor science and rational thought and, in the process, are sending eros into the unconscious. For many of them, doing so results in unembodied sex, which simply exacerbates loneliness.

The situation of Mary and her husband can be viewed in terms of the dynamics of animus–anima projection. Through her animus projection, Mary is unconsciously putting enormous pressure on her husband to perform in a certain way to meet her needs, which are in the emotional and spiritual realm, not in the biological realm. If she does not pull her projection back, she will resent him, as he will her, because it traps him into having to meet her expectations of being a certain way, thus enabling the animus-possessed woman. If Mary can engage in an ego–self dialogue, the positive animus can be developed within her as she begins to take back the projection. If John is unconscious of his anima projection, he will avoid her or get angry, because he believes that no matter what he does, it will never be enough to make her happy. This belief triggers his undeveloped anima, his inner feminine, and may feel like the emotional trap of his mother, whom he had to please as a child, as his father was absent much of the time.

The imprinting of imago

In the unconscious emotional brain, there is no discernment between mother or wife. The first love object, that of a mother, is experienced and imprinted as an important object, causing the child to feel completely dependent upon the object for his or her well-being. When John commits to Mary, in his unconscious, he will experience her as the same as his first love relationship, seeing her as an important object and responding to her in the same way he responded to his mother, whether that was trusting her or avoiding her. The coping skills John and Mary use as adults are the same coping skills they each used as young children with their parental love objects—coping skills that were used to defend against anxiety and/or shame.

This couple is in dire need of understanding the dynamics of anima and animus, which would open the doorway to the unconscious and could open the pathway to spiritual development. This avenue of instinctual energy is the first spark of the divine. Their relationship holds the *prima materia* for the uniting of the opposites. If the relationship can be made conscious, and the projections are recognized and retracted, albeit painfully, the development of the Self continues. If the projections remain, then the libido is blocked.

Often, libido may be blocked by the cunning silence of shame. Shame was in the Garden when the original choice was made to partake of knowledge. Shame appears in our earliest days of development as we give up our true self in order to develop a false self, hoping to please our parents, no matter the cost.

The withdrawing of projection

In the guided imagery exercise I conducted with Mary in the dialogue recorded above, she enters her imagination and first sees the child, observes what has happened, hears the feelings, and then rescues the child, meeting the child's need for protection and love. Guided imagery is necessary to take the child out of this situation, for if we do not rescue the child psychologically, the child remains in a victimized place. In the imaginative process with Mary, the child is rescued, and the feelings are heard and validated. This validation is important, as the unconscious reptilian brain does not know the difference between imagination and reality. If there is no intervention, then the repetition compulsion continues in the life of the adult, retraumatizing the child within. In going to this memory and giving the child what she needed, the energy that was trapped and blocked in Mary can now move and be responsive. In my opinion, Jung was teaching the neuroplasticity of the brain through active imagination, long before its recognition in the field of psychology today.

Turning to Mary's husband John's history, we can see how the two histories dance together. This physician's husband is an airline pilot. Both partners are driven and highly intelligent. So as not to feel vulnerable, both are overly responsible in their behavior toward each other, each taking care of the other with a high need to control. The intimacy they both long for is, in fact, what they most fear. Opposite fears of engulfment and abandonment are held simultaneously. In bed, they are asking the other to fill their needs or to make them feel loved.

John is the youngest of three children. His father was avoidant, and his mother was overbearing and controlling. We can see what attracted him to Mary, a strict and disciplined surgeon who can be overbearing in her expectations of performance. As the unconscious chooses the compensating factor in the other the picture of the two opposites is found. Being a pilot, he literally flies away in the face of any confrontation, which, for Mary, unconsciously echoes her father leaving her as a child. Mary experiences abandonment and then tries harder to gain his love, which triggers John's experience of an engulfing mother. Without consciousness of her need to feel safe and secure, she will orchestrate exactly how he is supposed to behave, thereby becoming the negative anima for him, ensuring that she will not get what she desires.

John experiences Mary's behavior as controlling and critical; thus, when she asks him for frontal penetration, he unconsciously fears being engulfed, as he did with his mother, whom he experienced as negative anima or devouring mother. Frontal penetration unconsciously scares him, and he flips her over so that, with Mary not looking at him, he can experience release from being controlled. On the other hand, Mary experiences the opposite when he flips her over, as it triggers her father leaving and being treated as being a piece of meat by her stepfather. What neither John nor Mary understands is that the unconscious is orchestrating this interaction, and no amount of sex toys or sex therapy is going to heal the problem. This is no longer about the other. To free them from the entrapment, their individual reclamation of unconscious material is required, and through that development, the energy for the creative process is freed.

Staples (2008) stated, "At a deep inner level sexuality and spirituality are reflected by the profane and the sacred, united by an underlying reality that acknowledges their interdependence. The truth is one has no meaning without the other." He claimed that understanding this interdependence requires becoming conscious. He further explained, "Consciousness is the capacity to differentiate.... We lose our paradisiacal innocence when we become aware of the opposites. We suffer for this capacity."

Paraphrasing a concept put forth by pastor Mark Driscoll and theologian Gary Breshears (2010, p. 349): *What I idolize, I will demonize*. This is a common theme I witness in the session. The biological aspect of desire brings us together, while at the same time, our unconscious woundedness attracts exactly who we need to play out the drama. According to Jung, "The unrelated human being lacks wholeness, for he can achieve wholeness only through the soul, and the soul cannot exist without its other side, which is always found in a 'You'" (1985, p. 244, para. 454). What in the beginning looks and feels like the divine soon goes to hell after we have mated and begin to commit. In the beginning, we idolize; later, we demonize. We attract the persona but come face-to-face with the shadow of ourselves as reflected in the other, or as Dr. Ribi suggested, "We marry our problems" (Personal Communication, January 2018). We impose upon the other all that is unresolved in ourselves. If the relationship does not promote the growth of each individual—even to risky, unpredictable places—it becomes a static or lifeless relationship. If one partner asks nothing of the relationship, there is no relatedness. In order to heal, we must make our wounds conscious and withdraw our projections from the beloved other, which can leave us in a difficult and lonely place.

One can see how the unconscious has orchestrated the very events that have ignited Mary's original woundedness. If physicians can learn about themselves in their marriage, that gift of presence or consciousness can be brought into awareness in both professional and personal relationships. The need to be seen and heard is a need we all have. One would think that this storyline is about sex; however, Jungian psychology takes a very different approach to healing. Sex is not the issue; it is simply the name of the drama being played out. In the case of Mary and John, sex reflects the deeper issue, which is a lack of nurturing, love, and protection.

Returning to the theme of shame, we find shame is often the dilemma in the human condition asking to be healed. There is no deeper shame than sexual shame. In the last four decades, I have listened to story after story from brilliant, successful physicians who had difficulty articulating their feelings or thoughts because of shame. These are not sick, dependent, addicted, weak, or otherwise pathologized physicians. These are physicians who are successful in their practices. They are dedicated to their marriages and family systems. Many of them have come from strong religious backgrounds. They come to my practice seeking wholeness and the unification of nature and spirit. They seek to reconcile the unconscious with the conscious and seek new ways to deal with their thoughts and feelings, not only within themselves but with others as well. Ideally, they come to understand that their longing is for the divine.

Unfortunately, physicians are taught that they do not need anything or anyone to help them, and believing that they can conduct their practice or their lives alone is problematic. This expectation sets in motion the process of shame, and in relation to this chapter, specifically sexual shame. No one can live in a perpetual state of innocence as in the Garden of Eden, where there is no shame. In reality, as life unfolds, shame takes one out of the innocent state of childhood, and perhaps, one of the deepest wounds to the Western human's psyche comes from sexual shame. We are not born with sexual shame; it is passed down through the personal as well as the collective unconscious.

If a medical doctor cannot talk about sex, who can? Sex is not ordinarily something clergy or teachers discuss, as they carry the shame as well. We are taught that if we feel sexual feelings for anyone other than our spouses, we are not okay. When we feel these absolutely normal feelings, we hide them. There are not good or bad feelings— they are simply feelings. We all have these feelings, whether we are conscious of them or not. In the case of sexual feelings, just because we feel them does not mean we must act on them.

Eros and logos

The split between eros and logos is evident in medical culture with regard to sexuality. The paradox is that physicians work on the body but are often terrified of their own bodies, so much so that often they act as if they do not have one. This splitting off from identification with the body means that sexual feelings go underground. The result is often sexual acting out, which is rampant in physician culture, as they desperately and unsuccessfully search for care and nurturing of the soul. This sexual acting out manifests as extramarital affairs as well as sexual addiction. In physician populations, sexually acting out seems to be directly related to the absence of eros in the logos-oriented world in which they are captured.

Through my many years of working with physicians, I have observed that they are less likely to act out sexually when they can acknowledge and manage the feeling side of themselves. I find that physicians avoid eros due to a perfectionism learned either through parental complexes or their medical training, or both. Whether the struggle for physicians in dealing with their sexuality manifests in their intimate relationships or in an unconscious acting out, they are in need of psychological deliverance. Western medical training has created an enormous psychological burden for physicians, and they are in dire need of relief as the kingdom of Western medicine declines. Change in the world of medicine is needed now more than ever. The words of W.B. Yeats (1997, 189–190) come to mind:

> *Turning and turning in the widening gyre*
>
> *The falcon cannot hear the falconer*
>
> *Things fall apart: the center cannot hold.*

References

Driscoll, M., & Breshears, G. (2010). *What Christians should believe*. Wheaton, IL: Crossway.

Jung, C.G. (1966). Medicine and psychotherapy. In H. Read, M. Fordham, G. Adler, & W. McGuire (Eds.), *The collected works of C. G. Jung: Vol. 16. The practice of psychotherapy*. R.F.C. Hull, (Trans.). Princeton, NJ: Princeton University Press.

Jung, C.G. (1985). The psychology of the transference. In H. Read, M. Fordham, G. Adler, & W. McGuire (Eds.), *The collected works of C. G. Jung: Vol. 16. The practice of psychotherapy*. R.F.C. Hull (Trans.). Princeton, NJ: Princeton University Press.

Jung, C.G. (1989). *Analytical psychology: Notes of the seminar given in 1925*. Princeton, NJ: Princeton University Press.

Staples, L. (2008). *Guilt with a twist: The Promethean way*. Sheridan, WY: Fisher King Press.

Yeats, W.B. (1921). *Michael Robartes and the dancer*. Wikisource [PD-old-80–1923]. https://en.wikisource.org/wiki/Michael_Robartes_and_the_Dancer/The_Second_Coming

Yeats, W. B. (1997). The second coming. In R.J., Finneran (Ed.), *Volume I: The Poems*. 2nd ed. New York, NY: Scribner.

Chapter 10

Suffering

> *And in the end, when the life went out of him and my hands could work no more, I left from that place into the night and wept—for myself, for life, for the tragedy of death's coming. Then I rose, and walking back to the suffering-house, forgot again my own wounds for the sake of healing theirs.*
>
> Anonymous ER doctor

The preceding passage is a story of life, which is both death and life. In my work, I frequently find physicians who have been taught only to focus on life, the first half of the life–death-life cycle. For the most part, the rest of the story has been unspoken or, better said, has been kept a secret. What happens to physicians when their hands can do no more? How do they learn to go into the darkness and weep? How do they learn to accept the tragedies or suffering of life? In the face of that darkness, how do they arise, not only for themselves but for others as well?

Individuation

This chapter recounts the wounds of suffering physicians that I have had the honor to witness. Like all of humanity, all physicians suffer. What is different in these accounts is how capable these men and women are in communicating their suffering. With the opportunity to give voice to their suffering and be heard, they no longer try to hide or feel shame about their wounds. They have brought the suffering into their conscious and no longer split it off or see it as a weakness. They have come to understand the second part of the story, which is death—not just mortal death but loss as well. Furthermore, the loss of hope and innocence points them toward individuation, which has the potential to bring them to a larger life.

Dr. Kildair, a retired surgeon, once told me what makes a physician go back into the "suffering-house" to suffer again. His explanation was that the physician is attached to outcome. When I asked him what he meant, he stated that when a physician loses a patient, he or she feels guilty. I

DOI: 10.4324/9781003144502-10

responded that this surprised me and asked what he meant. He said that if the patient dies, the physician feels responsible and guilty and that the suffering is an agony that is beyond words. He added,

> *You can't do this over and over, but, you know, if it's true, if the physician is responsible for the life he loses, then the opposite is true as well. When he is able to save a life, he feels just as good as he felt bad. It's all based on the outcome of the patient. The pendulum swings the other way. Until he learns he is neither the villain nor the hero, he will suffer.* (Personal Communication, 2016)

I asked if he meant a physician has to learn that the practice of medicine is not linear; instead it is circular, a cycle of both life and death, to which this surgeon replied, "He has to learn to not be attached to the outcome."

In a 12-step program, this position the surgeon described is called detachment, which does not mean aloofness or lack of caring. In depth psychology, not being attached to outcomes is called taking back our projections, meaning that one is no longer attached to something or someone for their value or well-being. In the program, this is understood as detachment. The thing one seeks cannot come from outside of oneself. Life's meaning is a function of the interiority of the personality and only comes through suffering. Life is a difficult, painful, yet holy process. When one sets the other person free, one is free. In the case of a physician, the patient is free to live or die. The physician recognizes something greater than themselves at work. Whether the patient lives or dies, the physician cannot define themselves by the outcome.

There must be something within the physician to help one decide for themselves what is true about who they are as a physician and the meaning of this experience with the patient that sometimes leads to suffering. Physicians' jobs are two-fold. They are to show up and "do" the very best that they can, and they have to be willing to "be" as fully present with their patients as they can. *Doing* the best one can is the masculine aspect of the personality, whereas being with the patient is relatedness, the feminine aspect of the personality. *Being* with the other is another way of bearing witness, of holding. When my discussion with the retired surgeon reached this point, he said to me clearly: "That is enough, that is all he can do, that is all that is humanly possible, that is enough. Then he is free to be a doctor."

The freedom of "enoughness"

This freedom occurs not because of the outcome of the patient but because of the holding of eros and logos by the physician. This physician experiences the meaning of "Physician, know thyself." This is the moment when the call of the physician becomes integrated into being the physician. When the physician needs nothing from the patient, not even for the patient to live, is a moment when the physician can do all he or she has been trained to do and to be all that he or she is called to be and may perhaps know for the first time that he or she is a doctor—a good doctor.

Dr. Jonas, a 72-year-old oncologist shared the following experience when I asked, "What happens to you when you do a surgery, and you know the outcome is bad? What happens when you see the patient and have to tell her you couldn't get all of the tumor?" I clarified that I was not asking what happens to the patient but wanted to know what happens inside of him as a physician. He responded,

> *When I leave her presence and the presence of the family, I pause for a moment in complete solitude, and I reflect on what has just happened. I am able to be with myself, alone for a brief moment. It sometimes just feels bittersweet. I am in that moment in between and remember that I cared and took care of my patient the best I could. When I go home and listen to music and contemplate that what I did with a particular patient is not only from what I learned from a book but what I know from experience. I remind myself that I have done everything I could do to save her life. I was well-trained as a surgeon, and no one could have done more than I did, and that is enough. That is all I can do. That has to be enough.* (Personal Communication, 2016)

I asked if he would think of her as he leaves her care, and he responded that, in fact, he would and added that for him it is a kind of acceptance. I asked him what he would feel; he responded, "It's a kind of acceptance. You see, the physician goes through the grief stages just like the patient and the family. It doesn't just happen when the patient dies, but when I know there is loss. There is sadness." When I asked if he cried, he replied: "Sometimes I do, and sometimes I don't. Not all patients are the same." I then asked him, if he experienced loss or sadness, would he talk to anyone about those feelings, and he stated that he would not. When I asked him, "What do you do with those feelings?" he asked what I meant. I clarified by asking him whether he denied his feelings and moved on to the next patient or paused and worked with the longings of his soul to acknowledge his own feelings. He replied, "Sometimes I think about the family, the children, the kids, the husband, but no I don't talk about it. All of those feelings just go inside of me, and I guess I just push them down."

It is in regard to pushing down the feelings Dr. Jonas described that I believe analytical psychology offers a new direction for the physician. Rather than denying the feeling, physicians must learn that the feeling itself is healing, even if it is difficult or painful. Their feelings tell physicians what they value and what is important to them. Not to honor this aspect of the personality of the physician is costly in terms of psychological and physical health, as discussed previously. I believe the feeling aspect of the physician invites eros into the relationship with the self and the other, even if it means suffering. The ability to hold suffering and the unknown outcome is to be with that process. This is a uniting principle of the psyche. The positive feminine is the receptacle of love or matter; the positive masculine is the spirit that goes into the eternal unknown in search of meaning. The Self, in Jung's conception, is the totality of the conscious and unconscious psyche, which can never be fully understood. In his book *Symbols of Transformation* (1967), Jung described the Self, as a symbol of wholeness, a *coincidentia oppositorum*, the coming together of the opposites and therefore containing light and dark simultaneously. Jung found this phenomenon expressed in the inner experience of the individual.

It is those individual experiences that offer the invitation for the physician to begin or continue the individuation process. To be individuated is to be able to let the masculine and feminine energies work together. When one side is not split off, and ego is strong enough, the container of the self holds them together and something new emerges. When asked why they suppress their feelings, the common retort is to survive, as they do not know another way to cope with their feelings. Isolating themselves from the patient and separating themselves from their own feelings leaves the experience one-sided, thereby viewing the patient as an object to be acted upon. If the patient is seen merely as something to be cured, a product of sorts, that is patriarchal thinking focusing on outcome, which strips the soul's inner life, and according to Jung, this brings no healing for the patient nor the physician. I propose that before we can begin to think about changing the structure of medicine as a business, time and energy must be devoted to teaching the physician to connect with their humanity. I think this is what Dr. Jonas is telling us. He is not laying out four basic rules to becoming a better physician; he is telling us to accept the physician with his or her own limitations. This doctor is telling us that when he is able to hold the patient in his heart and to hold himself and his knowing of himself, he is essentially saying, "I know who I am and this knowing tells me I am valuable, not just my persona, but also as a human being." He is saying that because he can value himself and know what is true for him, he is then free to be a good physician regardless of outcome. When this man chooses to be alone with himself, he offers the opportunity for soul and imagination to come together. His conscious feminine aspect opens up the groundwork for creativity, generated by the penetrating conscious masculine. In having no control over the outcome, by simply being present, he is free to experience being fully alive as a physician.

This physician's story combines experience with knowledge, connecting body with spirit, thus creating soul. Knowing him, I said that I suspected that after difficult experiences with patients he would go home and listen to music. He responded: "Yes, music comforts me." Both Dr. Kildair and Dr. Jonas's accounts above have a commonality. Both physicians are in their 70s and possess the ability to define enoughness that seems to have become an imperative in accepting themselves as physicians. Some of the patients will live and some will die. It seems the physician's task is to hold both mysteries—life and death. Yet, it is not the older physicians who are killing themselves literally and metaphorically. It is the young medical residents or clinicians in their practice of medicine who are most at risk and vulnerable. How do we help them find the answers that these two mature physicians have found? How do we help them hold the tension of the opposites?

The pain of the wounded healer

When one is able to stand alone, separate from the collective, and able to define for oneself who one is and not be defined by the other, then individuation is in process. As one stands in the middle of life and death, feeling the tension, one has the opening to begin to experience the movement of life. Holding the tension of these opposites can move one to a place of creation in which something is born with each death, and with each birth there is also a death; both are part of the circular nature of life. Is this not the symbol of the Uroboros, the snake who is eating its tail, completing the life-death-life cycle? Perhaps the sacred or the holiness of life must be experienced as the wholeness of life.

Rather than waging war when a physician cannot save a life, let the physician learn how the conscious feminine depends on recognition by the masculine, just as the masculine depends on being seen by the feminine. Physicians and patients simply need each other in the inner as well as in the outer world. Let us hold the tensions between the opposites without negating either one. This is not an either-or way of being but rather both-and. The worlds of the physician and the patient are not exclusive but rather inclusive of each other.

In the field of medicine in the United States, in 1989, a fairly new ceremony originated called the white coat ceremony. Physicians are asked to represent themselves as scientists by putting on the most recognizable symbol of the scientist—the white laboratory coat. This white coat is symbolic of their consciousness of medicine as science; however, another meaning placed upon this symbol of science and rationality is that of the serpent wrapped around a staff, the symbol of Asclepius, the god of medicine. Notably, this symbol holds the duality of life, the irrational, or the mystery of life. Jung denoted that the serpent is not only an animal but also a magical animal and presupposed that hardly anyone is neutral in relation to snakes (Jung, 1984). Just as horses and monkeys have instinctive snake phobias, so do humans. According to Jung, as an animal, the snake symbolizes something unconscious, instinctual; the snake shows the way to the hidden treasure, or is the guardian of the treasure, yet the serpent is symbolic of healing. The serpent holds both life and death. Jung pointed out that Philo of Alexandria, impressed with the serpent's ability to rejuvenate itself through the shedding of its skin as well as its ability to kill and cure (which Jung saw as indicative of the positive and negative cosmic powers that rule the world), deemed it the "most spiritual of animals" According to Jungian analyst Joseph Henderson (1964),

> Perhaps the commonest dream symbol of transcendence is the snake, represented by the therapeutic symbol of the Roman god of medicine Asclepius, which has survived into modern times as a sign of the medical profession. This was originally a non-poisonous tree snake; as we see it coiled around the staff of the healing god, it seems to embody a kind of mediation between earth and heaven.

Jung (1960), however, also clarified that "this serpent does not represent 'reason' or anything approaching it, but rather symbolizes a peculiar autonomous mind which can possess one completely, a spirit of revelation which gives us (intuitions)." What does this say to the physician?

The physician as both god and human must come to see suffering as a part of life as well as a part of his or her calling, long before being able cognitively to understand the meaning of the call. Physicians own it, or perhaps they might more correctly say the call owns them. They speak of sacrifice more readily than they do of suffering; however, the sacrifices they make are a part of their suffering, though sacrifice and suffering are not the same thing. The verb *to suffer* comes from the Latin word *suffer*, meaning "to hold up, carry, to bear, to endure," whereas the root word for *sacrifice* comes from the Latin *sacer* meaning "holy," thus an offering to make sacred or holy. This begs the question: can suffering have holy meaning, or must we suffer and endure without meaning?

I asked one of the physician groups, whose ages range from 35 to 50, what the most difficult thing was about being a physician. The majority of them said something like "I can't just turn it off. When I go home, I take the patient home with me, wherever I am, I just can't turn it off." When I shared with them the accounts of the physicians above, they asked, "What happens to you when you don't do the best you could do?", and "What happens when you operated and you were too tired to make the best decisions?", "What happens when you failed to read a chart correctly and it affects the whole family?" I then asked a 35-year-old OB-Gyn physician, who had responded with such a question, to explain what she was talking about. Through her tears, she told me the following story:

> I was pregnant, due the next month. I was trying to get all my patients seen before I left, and I was in a hurry. This woman [patient] had asked me for a genetic workup. I followed through and arranged for the testing. When the results came back, I checked the results, charted them and never told the expectant mom. Six months later, she gave birth to a genetic

disordered child that will change her and her family's life forever. It wasn't the best I could do. I caused enormous pain that won't get better. This child will live a full life of being disabled, and this family, this mom and dad requested this particular test so this wouldn't have happened. How can I accept that as the best I can do? (Personal Communication, September 2017)

The entire group was silent. I asked this physician if she could picture herself on that day the results came in, charting them but not making the phone call to the mom. I asked her if she could see herself at her desk with the results in her hand, putting them in the chart. She replied that she could. I then asked if she could see herself in the delivery room when the baby was born and knowing immediately there was a defect. She replied yes. I then asked if she, the physician sitting here before me now, was telling me clearly that she made a mistake. Again, she replied yes and that she could not correct it. I agreed with her, as the baby had been born. I then asked what happened that day of the baby's birth. She replied,

I went immediately to the office to look at their chart. I couldn't believe that I had missed it. Yet there it was, a positive result for translocation trisomy 21, resulting in Down syndrome. I then went to the patient's room and told them I had it in their chart. It was my mistake and I apologized. We all cried. I wondered if they were going to sue me? They still could.

I reaffirmed aloud that she had made a mistake and asked her what she might do with that part of her. Was she not as valid as the physician sitting before me now, not still the same person, all of her? Yes, the emotions of regret and sadness, guilt, and perhaps fear of a lawsuit were there. Could she hold those emotions and feel them? Could she hold both sides of herself—her oath asking to do no harm and her reality of facing the harm she had done, even though unintentional? Could she hold these opposites? Could she stand to feel these feelings? I followed these questions with this statement:

That, my dear, is your task. Those older physicians whose accounts I shared with you talked about the best they could do, but they did not talk about perfection. They spoke of acceptance of their limits. It seems to me you are being asked to separate from your collective medical authority bringing your own sense of self, all of yourself, into consciousness. I am speaking of guilt. What will you do with this guilt to enlarge your life, not to reduce it to the dualistic thinking of medical school?

The room was quiet. For they all knew at some level that what she was experiencing in that moment would also be their experience. In his book

Mysterium Coniunctionis (1963), Jung wrote about the different roles of guilt, saying that guilt and life are connected to each other in the development of human consciousness. If the physician is to become conscious and individuated, then guilt in its many forms must be addressed, for "guilt is the price we must pay for the privilege of experiencing life as a human" (Pennington & Staples, 2011).

Suffering and sacrifice and serpents

Drawing on Staples' (2008) discussion of society's different views of guilt, I want to describe briefly two that are relevant to this discussion. The first, we learned as young children when we made choices that violated the authoritarian rules that were placed upon us—in other words, this is a violation of the other. A healthy response to this type of guilt is to own our behavior and to make amends to the party we have offended, intentional or not, as was the scenario in the story of the baby with Down syndrome. This type of guilt is important in the maintenance of conventional life. This conventional guilt keeps us within boundaries deemed acceptable and helps us resist doing things that would bring harm to our individual and collective interest.

The second kind of guilt comes from a violation not of the community but of the self. Staples referred to this as *Promethean guilt*. He recounted the ancient myth of Prometheus stealing fire from the gods and making it available for use by humans. Prometheus suffered for his sin. Zeus had him chained to a rock where an eagle pecked and tore daily at his liver; however, human society would have suffered if he had not committed this violation. This type of guilt suggests the importance of "sinning" and incurring guilt in order to obtain needed but forbidden things. One cannot respond to these types of guilt in the same way because, as Staples (2008) stated, "the Promethean spirit that is supported by an obstinate and irreverent insolence toward authority is informed by a love of freedom."

Jung was clear that there is a high and demanding price to be paid for guilt (and, I propose, for shame, as discussed later in this chapter), when one gives up conventional life and travels the path of individuation. In the following passages, Jung also directed us to a way this guilt might be redeemed:

[The individuating person]... must offer a ransom in place of himself, that is, he must bring forth values, which are an equivalent substitute for his absence in the collective, personal sphere. (1976, p. 451, para. 1095)

The individual is obligated by the collective demands to purchase his individuation at the cost of an equivalent work for the benefit of society. (p. 452, para. 1099)

As Staples (2008) recounted, "in Greek mythology, Prometheus went far away to where the gods lived, stole fire, and brought it back. He offended the gods and incurred guilt and punishment for his deed, but his guilty deed brought great benefit to mankind." Examples of this type of deed could be "Rosa Parks, Susan B Anthony, Galileo, and Socrates," just to name a few. Jesus and his followers also had to be willing to be seen as "heretics" and living on the outside. This is close to the feeling of shame, closely akin to guilt. These people were not forbearers of the existing order. "They brought fresh new ideas to the world and they suffered for it" (Staples, 2008). When such a demand is made by Psyche upon the individual, there is a cost for going there, and likewise there is a cost for not going there.

Promethean guilt or healthy guilt is the guilt that we feel when we follow the path of individuation, which leads us outside of the collective or conventional pattern of life. The human psyche is a self-regulating system that maintains its equilibrium throughout compensatory processes: for example, when the ego becomes too one-sidedly extraverted, the self creates a compensatory urge toward its opposite, introversion. When one opposite becomes so dominant that the other opposite's existence is threatened, the self-attempts to restore balance by weakening the stronger or strengthening the weaker. The individuated physician is able to hold the desire for perfection and yet also able to hold the imperfection of limitations and, likewise, the feeling of sexual attraction to a patient and, at the opposite end, the ability to hold the feeling and not act on it. The psychological process of bringing these opposites together without sending something away is the transcendent function, which holds the tensions of the two opposites until a third thing appears. Referring to Jung's theory, Staples (2008) wrote, "As the ego becomes increasingly capable of containing both opposites simultaneously, it comes increasingly to be a more accurate reflection of the self, the archetype of wholeness and totality."

This book is about the wholeness of the physicians' humanity, not only the hero but also the villain and the scapegoat. How do they begin to own these other parts of themselves, the parts that are not perfect and can hurt others? As I posited before, how do we help the younger physician gain the capacity to hold both the positive and negative aspects of the self? I believe this is done by talking with them and bringing the light into the dark places, inviting them to make the shadow they fear conscious. I am reminded of a poem by Persian poet Jalāl āl-dīn Rumi (1995):

The Guest House

This being human is a guest house.
Every morning a new arrival.
A joy, a depression, a meanness,
Some momentary awareness comes
As an unexpected visitor.
Welcome and entertain them all!
Even if they are a crowd of sorrows,

Who violently sweep your house empty of its furniture,
Still, treat each guest honorably.
He may be clearing you out
For some new delight.
The dark though, the shame, the malice,
Meet them at the door laughing and invite them in.
Be grateful for whatever comes.
Because each has been sent
As a guide from beyond.

The following is a story of a physician's shame. A young female, a chief resident in her third year of residency in medical school, met with me four months prior to her graduation. She came to see me because she was suicidal, with a plan to cut her femoral artery. She saw no choices but only entrapment—the entrapment of shame. She did not yet know there was an alternative way of dealing with shame. A glimpse into her history revealed a child on the receiving end of her parental complexes.

She experienced early feelings of abandonment by her mother and, as a child, became her father's confidant and was made aware of the affairs in which her father had engaged. Imprinted in her unconscious was the critical and aloof voice of mother and the unavailability of a father who appeared to be there for her but, in actuality, was there for his emotional needs to be met by her. She came to understand that no matter how good she was, she could never be enough, as a child is unable to meet the emotional needs of the parent. Striving to receive love and approval, she excelled academically, with little social interaction in her adolescent years.

The cunning silence of shame

The unconscious is relentless in moving one to wholeness and healing, as reflected in the experiences of this woman in her young medical career. As her story unfolded, she revealed that she had become involved in destructive sexual behavior with her attending physician. He was known for his sexual harassment in this particular medical school and had been previously reported to administration. The imago seemed to fit. Here was the male authority figure posing as loving and interested, who, in reality, was only there to exploit this young naive student. The mother role was played out by a woman who was head of the department, to whom the young resident went for help. The department chair's response was "We have to protect the program and the school. You told me this has been going on for ten months." The young woman commented to me,

I get why people don't tell. You get blamed. In the past couple of weeks
there have been three attempted suicides: two completions and one brain

dead. This is what I am going to be known for in residency. I am asked, "Is this how you got to be chief, by sleeping with Dr. X? (Personal communication, June 2017)

This hospital harbored a shame-based system that was ruled by secrecy and power. This young woman's superior had power over her and used her naiveté for his gain. The product was the shame which she had identified as her own. It was helpful for her to learn that the unconscious was asking for something *in her* to die, but it was not asking her to die. What needed to die was her repeated pattern of negative self-talk and her ignorance of protective choices, which she had inherited from her parents. The secrets of the medical school that she carried along with her shame needed to die, not her.

The following narratives reflect different aspects of shame and how it is often experienced in the medical community. Shame is universal. Shame is that feeling washing over us to tell us we feel small, flawed, never good enough, and we do not want anyone to know we are feeling it. We can do one of two things with shame. We can either identify it and learn to work with it, transforming shame into the gift of compassion, first, for ourselves and then the other. Alternatively, we can deny it and insulate ourselves with the wall of arrogance often called aloofness, becoming smaller in our hiddenness. The former way of dealing with shame invites relationship, whereas the latter destroys relationship; both are rooted in shame. Shame refers to humiliation so painful, embarrassment so deep, and such a sense of being completely diminished that one may feel invisible. Shame involves the entire self and self-worth of a human being. Shame is an inner sense of being less than, inferior, inadequate, or insufficient as a person; however, this is the self-judging the self. Sustained shame creates an ongoing premise: "If others really knew me, they would find me lacking."

This shame originates in our identity development influenced by how our caregivers and authority figures view and treat us. Shame prevails in institutions, and the world of medicine is in no way exempt. The following two accounts relate to shame in medicine. Both accounts speak to a broken medical system in dire need of a new container. Metaphorically speaking, a new wineskin is necessary as the old wineskin can no longer contain the wine. As wine is a spirit, it is notable that the Latin word for *spirit* is *spiritus*. Like an old wineskin, the spirit of medicine can no longer be contained in such a restricted and limited form. A new container is called for—a container large enough to hold not only the physical and intellectual aspects of medicine but also the emotional and spiritual components. The process of letting go of the old is painful, but the predominantly patriarchal medical system, in which productivity is the main focus, is no longer working for either the physician or the patient, as these narratives attest.

An OB-Gyn physician in his 50s told me the following story:

I had known this patient a long time. She shared with me a level of grace I had not experienced before nor have I since. Pregnant with her second child, I wanted her to have amniocentesis because of her age. I may have even talked her into it. I was young and full of myself. I thought I was pretty good and counseled her to have the amniocentesis [an invasive procedure that carries the risk of causing miscarriage].

On the day of the procedure, I thought all went well. However, when she called me ten days later, I heard the fear in her voice as she explained she was leaking fluid and running a fever. I asked her to meet me at the hospital, even though I wasn't on call. With heaviness and dread, I did a sonogram. The results validated that her pregnancy was no longer viable. Her perfectly normal baby was lost. I lost this pregnancy for her and felt bad for a very long time. I expected a records request the next day, and my partners said she would probably sue me. She did not. She stuck with me as a patient. In fact, I delivered her next baby, and last week, I did her hysterectomy. I cared about her. I cared about what happened and felt embarrassed and ashamed. I felt helpless to make things better. There is no worse feeling for a doctor. I recall sitting with her after her sonogram trying to deal with the emotions between us. I felt full of sadness. (Personal Communication, 2017)

As the physician told this story, his legs were crossed, his foot was moving rapidly, and his breathing was shallow. He stopped speaking several times before completing his story. I asked him what he was feeling, and he replied that he was feeling very sad. He said,

She had every right to be mad at me, but she never expressed that. Instead, when I apologized, we both wept quietly. She said, "These things happen. I feel bad for you and it's not your fault. I trust you and love you, and I'm not going to leave you." Sometime afterward, she moved away with her family. I missed her. She called not long ago to tell me she was moving back. Her OB-Gyn in the city where she lived had recommended a hysterectomy. She was calling for a second opinion and said she wanted to wait until the family move was completed and that she wanted me to do the surgery. I agreed.

Somehow, she is more than a patient in a way I don't fully understand. I have to be careful not to cross boundaries. I sense she has an affinity for me as more than just a doctor. After the move, she came to see me and seemed truly interested in me and my boys, but not in a seductive way. She seemed to see my care and concern and to see me for who I really am.

When she lost her baby, I didn't try to hide my emotion. I know she saw my tears and sensed the heaviness in my heart. She had every right to be angry

with me; however, she didn't use my vulnerability against me. I couldn't imagine ever feeling vulnerable, but I did. I just sat with her that day, and she saw me, and I her. I have thought a lot about this experience. For me it was a rare moment in my life when I felt seen. It was especially meaningful coming from someone who didn't seem to need anything from me. Instead, she simply needed me to be her doctor, not God. She helped me by asking questions about who I am and what I do. It felt like one of those rare moments when you love someone. We both felt it—but nothing inappropriate had to happen. We could just hold it there in that moment, not only 15 years ago, but today as well. Sometimes when she asks things about my life, I am perplexed. I'm not used to people asking about me. Yet when she hugs me, I am afraid of those feelings.

When I asked, "Feelings?" he continued, telling me how he also takes care of her mother. I reminded him he was expressing a thought, not a feeling. "What were the feelings you were afraid of?" I asked. "I guess they are feelings that I care about her.", he answered. I asked, "Feelings of warmth?" "Yes," he replied.

I reminded him that medical schools disavow feeling just as our culture sexualizes the love emotion simply because we don't know what to do with those feelings. He continued: "Sometimes I am afraid to trust these feelings." I asked him what he was afraid of. Was he afraid of betraying himself and his values? His response was "No, but you know my history—I have trusted women who have hurt me." I asked him if he was afraid of being hurt, but a more relevant question might have been "Do you know how to deal with the hurt that may come when we allow ourselves to be vulnerable?"

I said to him, "She trusts you and you know that. Perhaps you love her enough to hold your boundary as a physician—a balance of logos and eros. You didn't send the feelings away nor did you act inappropriately. These feelings occur. Feelings are not good or bad. Your job is to know they are there, identify them, and then behave in a way that is congruent with your calling as a physician."

The gift of empathy for physicians and patients

Yes, there is an unconscious connection that occurs, and this can be experienced as healing for both the physician and the patient. A physician can love his or her patient, and the patient can love the physician. Why do we have to pathologize this? We don't. While it is a vulnerable place, it is not problematic when one knows himself or herself. It's not just knowing diagnostic skills or surgery—it's understanding the relational skill of being with someone in their suffering. This can only come when a physician learns to deal with his or her own suffering rather than denying it. It requires a willingness to enter into the very thing one is most afraid of—emotional pain. When a physician can identify his or her feelings and work with them, this vulnerability can be transformed into the gift of empathy. This allows an appropriate and meaningful connection to occur and honors the sacredness inherent in the practice of medicine.

The OB-Gyn physician continued: "This story takes me back to junior high school. I was in science class and sat next to Kelly Jones. Kelly was the prettiest girl I had ever seen. She was smart, too, and I got to sit next to her. I thought we were friends and looked forward to talking with her in class. After a couple of months, I asked Kelly if she would go steady with me. She laughed and said, 'I would never go steady with you.' I was silenced for the rest of the year and understand now this was the feeling of shame. I felt helpless and knew I couldn't take it back. I took a risk, and it didn't work out well. It taught me I wasn't good enough."

I responded, "No, my friend, it didn't teach you weren't good enough—you already believed that. This was just a validation. What you weren't good at was how to deal with the emotional pain of rejection. You made up that if you were good at reading her mind, you wouldn't have asked her to go steady and this painful event would have never happened."

He said, "I wasn't good at reading people's feelings—it was awful."

I asked, "What did you do? Did you talk to anyone about it?"

"No," he said, "I didn't want anyone to know about it—I just packaged it up and buried it."

Here, shame raised its ugly head. He knew how to reject himself as well as his vulnerability, and yet he had no one to help him navigate the emotional waters. How can someone that young know how to respond to shame, much less understand how it developed, or how to respond to it in a healthy way? When shame overtakes us, it hurts, and we just want it to go away. Most often we utilize two coping skills: avoid or please. We learn these skills as children, but they are ineffective and inhumane in adulthood if we do not make them conscious. As adults, we would not wear the shoes of a five-year-old, yet we will use these archaic defenses that no longer serve us.

Unwelcome inheritance

Both the story of this physician's experience with his patient and the story of his rejection by his junior high classmate have a connection to his family of origin. He was the youngest of three, with a father who was absent due to work. He thus became aligned with his wheelchair-bound mother, who suffered from multiple sclerosis. Though it was unspoken, he understood that his job was to take care of his mother and make her happy. This situation was the source of his original wounding. The child introjects the suffering mother unconsciously into his or her young developing psyche, whose ego is not developed to defend against it. A child cannot meet the emotional needs of an adult and projecting them onto a child is inappropriate.

Neither of the physician's parents was bad or mean; they were simply unconscious and unaware of the harm the family dynamic created in the imprinting of their young son. Notably, as a young boy, he was praised for how well he cared for his mother. Only years later did he come to believe he was never going to be enough for his mother or any woman who looked to him to make her happy.

In this family system, by his absence, the father silently colluded with the mother. The well-being of the mother was handed down to the child. This also created in the young boy a hunger for his father—someone who would protect him from what the physician called "too much mother" and would teach him that he already had inside of him everything he needed to make his way in the world. He needed a male advocate to teach him he was enough. Later in life, he realized that his father had not taught him how to deal with women but instead had unconsciously instilled in him how to be gone, how to work, and how to feel guilty or ashamed when he could not make a woman happy. This belief system continued into adulthood, no matter how successful the physician became. He learned to manage his anxiety and fear of being engulfed by pleasing people and taking care of others. Neither enlarged his life.

Unfortunately for him, the childhood neural pathways created in childhood continued to be played over and over in his unconscious emotional brain with a type of repetition compulsion. In the story of rejection by the girl in junior high. the outward experience validates the inner belief created much earlier in his life— "I am not enough." Left unattended, these unconscious belief patterns are reactivated when one deals with emotional pain in adulthood, as evidenced in the adult life of this physician. If the unconscious need to be enough and thereby gain parental approval and love is not made conscious and processed, the physician can become dependent upon needing the approval of the patient, which can put the physician in harm's way. The skill of taking care of people provided an outward, temporary salve to the deep inner conflict in relation to his own value and worthiness.

As an adult, this bright and deeply feeling man entered the profession of medicine, which seemed fitting, given his desire to care for others and his ability to achieve. He married after medical school and joined a private practice, which was followed by the birth of twin boys. Within two years of their births, his wife was diagnosed with breast cancer, and one of the boys developed leukemia, which required a bone marrow transplant. His brother became the donor. After the transplant, a year later, the physician's wife had a recurrence of breast cancer. His life became a blur of taking care of everyone but himself—an unconscious repetition of the use of coping mechanisms developed in childhood. Burying his own needs and working harder to take care of others were the makings of an inevitable crisis.

Needless to say, from a very young age this physician did not know how to deal with emotional pain outside of taking care of other people. Though this early learning set the stage for the making of a great physician, it also set the stage for relationship difficulties in adulthood. This early patterning also explains how taken aback this physician was when his patient accepted him rather than sue him when she lost her baby. He was so struck by her not needing anything from him except just to be her doctor. Adding to his surprise was that someone could love him when he did not feel lovable. He did not understand that it was his birthright to be loved by another being not just for what he could do for that person.

This man's need to be seen and heard was not met by his mother, which developed in him a negative mother complex. This experience led him to be attracted to needy women. He found that no matter how hard he tried, he would never be enough to take care of them. In fact, he married a woman who wanted him to take care of her. Over the years, he asked her to grow, to have a life of her own, without focusing exclusively on him. Unfortunately, she was unable to risk living her own separate life interdependently with his. When the stress became unbearable and the burden too heavy, he had an affair. Over time and through suffering, he realized the affair was not about sex or love but was instead a desperate attempt to find temporary relief. This relationship was brutal and painful and ended with the physician experiencing enormous shame and self-doubt. For the first time in his life, he came face to face with his childhood woundedness and the need to be loved in the way he needed as a child. For the adult, this could no longer be met by a woman. What he was searching for now could only be found within himself as he learned how to parent the child within.

Through this crisis, the physician began to see the beauty of his own life. While he still struggled with the affair, he also understood the necessity of his divorce that followed, though he wished he had addressed it in a more constructive way. In the physician's group, when I asked him where he might have learned the coping skill of avoidance, the room was silent. The unfinished business of the father had become the business of the adult child, signifying a negative father complex as well. The physician's first attempt at dealing with shame was to achieve. If he excelled, he could avoid temporarily feeling shame, so he had gotten a good education, chosen a respected profession, and married a beautiful woman only to find out, again, that for him, nothing was more painful than disappointing the other.

Over time, the physician came to understand that the lack of boundaries in the parental dyad had set him up to feel the emotions of anxiety and shame. His father unconsciously taught him how to avoid conflict through lack of boundary setting, while his mother leaned on him to meet her emotional needs. What was unexpected, however, was that when these dynamics were made conscious, old attitudes that no longer served the Self would begin to die so that new attitudes could be put in place. Although it took what initially seemed like a crisis, by understanding the context of his childhood development, he began to learn how to mother and father himself. The crisis may have actually initiated the process of individuation for this physician. This is the highest psychological calling: to come home to one's self, only to find joy and beauty within, which then also impacts community. For this physician, the process of coming home to himself is well under way.

References

Henderson, J. (1964). Ancient myths and modern man. In C.G. Jung & M.-L. von Franz (Eds.), *Man and his symbols*. London, England: Aldus Books.

Jung, C.G. (1976). Adaptation, individuation, collectivity. In H. Read, M. Fordham, G. Adler, & W. McGuire (Eds.), *The collected works of C. G. Jung: Vol. 18. The symbolic life*. Princeton, NJ: Princeton University Press.

Jung, C.G. (1984). *Dream analysis: Notes of the seminar given in 1928–1930*. In W. McGuire (Ed.). Princeton, NJ: Princeton University Press.

Jung, C.G. (1960). *Modern psychology: Notes on lectures given at the Eidgenossische Technische Hochschule, Zurich: alchemy, vols. 1 & 2*. In B. Hannah (Ed.). E. Welsh (Trans.). Zurich, Switzerland: Schippert.

Jung, C.G. (1967). *The collected works of C. G. Jung: Vol. 5. Symbols of transformation*. H. Read, M. Fordham, G. Adler, & W. McGuire (Eds.). R.F.C. Hull (Trans.). Princeton, NJ. Princeton University Press.

Jung, C.G. (1963). *The collected works of C. G. Jung: Vol. 14. Mysterium coniunctionis*. H. Read, M. Fordham, G. Adler, & W. McGuire (Eds.). R.F.C. Hull (Trans.). Princeton, NJ. Princeton University Press.

Pennington, Nancy C., & Staples, Lawrence H. (2011). *The guilt cure*. Sheridan, WY: Fisher King Press.

Rumi, J.a.-d. (1995). The Essential Rumi (Expanded ed.). (C. Barks, Trans.). San Francisco, CA: Harper San Francisco.

Staples, L. (2008). *Guilt with a twist: The Promethean Way*. Sheridan, WY: Fisher King Press.

Chapter 11

A mythic monster named shame

Shame is the only emotion we are not born with. We learn shame. It is experienced in our very first relationships leaving an imprint that haunts the soul and yearns for redemption. We experience shame when we haven't been able to be the person we wanted people to think we are.

Personal Communication, 2016

The Chinese say that the dragon possesses the power of metamorphosis and the gift of rendering itself invisible. Shame's invisibility is powerful; yet, the invisible in life is what we long to know intimately (Fossum & Mason, 1989). When we experience the emotion of shame, we experience humiliation, embarrassment, and a sense of diminishment. Shame involves the entire self and self-worth of a human being. It is the self judging the self. Yet in this very moment of judging we long to be known, not for who we present ourselves to be but who we authentically are.

Shame: Who bears this burden?

This story was told by a woman who, at age 14, was seriously injured in a horrific car accident. When the family car was hit by a drunk driver, she was thrown from the burning car. Her mother and sister perished. She recounted the aftermath of this tragedy:

I was 14 years old. I had just survived an automobile accident that took the lives of my 41-year-old mother and my sister, who was 17. I sustained mostly third-degree burns over 56 percent of my body. I was being treated in the best burn center closest to where we lived, which was also a teaching hospital. The treatment of burn injuries can be horrific, or more so than the actual catastrophe that caused the burns. The daily "takings" that involved debriding the dead tissue were always a dreaded time for me.

One specific morning, I was in the tank enduring the procedure when a doctor entered the treatment room. He swiftly and coldly asked if it would

DOI: 10.4324/9781003144502-11

be alright for several student doctors to observe my treatment. They all came through the door at the exact same time as the lead physician had come in, which indicated that compliance was expected. I barely had time to see if my nude body was covered [it was, by a small towel]. I felt overwhelmed. Here I was, an innocent, pubescent, 14-year-old girl, enduring excruciating physical pain, managing the emotional weight of uncertainty of survival from my injuries, while at the same time grieving the tremendous loss of my mother and sister. I was raw and vulnerable like never before or since. The group of six young, handsome male student doctors entered my treatment room, watching my naked body being debrided, full of anticipation and quest for knowledge. Their energy and enthusiasm disregarded the gravity of my condition. Not one of those men looked me in the eye, introduced themselves, or thanked me for allowing them the opportunity to observe my state. I felt violated by their power yet indebted to their power at the same time. I realized they needed this experience to improve their medical skill, but acquiring this knowledge at the expense of contributing to a young girl's feelings of victimization was never considered.

The invisible

Lying there, I watched them explore my wounds with their eyes. I could not make out their words to each other. I mentally returned to the deep place within myself—a place that I already knew too well. The place where I was alone with my pain, grief, shame, fear, and misery. My spirit and soul were invisible in that room with a half-dozen doctors and two nurses. They did not see my personal essence; they only saw the wounds inflicted upon me in the car accident. I wonder what small changes in behavior these professionals could have made that would have empowered me, instead of stripping me of my dignity and self-worth.

I believe a few simple changes in their approach could have made all the difference. They could have taken the time to see me while I was still in my hospital room, still decent, and in the place that I was most familiar with and which felt safest to me at the time. They could have looked me in the eye and each told me his name and asked mine. We could have shared a moment of conversation. Maybe we would have discovered some common-alities and learned a bit about each other. Maybe I would have felt seen as a person, not just as my wounds. I wonder how differently I would recall this encounter if I had felt included in this process instead of treated like an outsider. (Personal Communication, August 2017)

"Did you think these physicians were calloused?" I asked her. She replied, "No," and sighed, "I don't know what they were." I inquired, "Did you feel valued by them?" She responded, "Only my injuries. Only my injuries. They didn't deal with me." Susan continued to reflect: "That felt awful. I remember thinking if I was here because they were the best, and they didn't know what to do with me, who was going to take care of me? I was terrified, and I don't know if it was because they thought I was going to die. I didn't know if they hadn't seen anybody burned this bad, I remember thinking I was too much for them."

"Is that what you made up when no information was given to you?" I asked. (This can touch original beliefs of a child which may be "my needs are too much.") "Yes," she answered. "I remember hearing in the ambulance that they were taking me to the hospital near the accident site but they couldn't handle me, and I was transported to a larger hospital in a near by city. I just remember thinking and wondering, *'Who can deal with me?'*"

Fear-based shame is evidenced in this conversation going on inside of Susan's head, her inner dialogue. The silence regarding her condition and the destination only validated her historical, unconscious, questioning beliefs. For the patient, the aloofness, arrogance, heartbreak, or whatever motivated the physicians' silence was hurtful. Was their attitude masking the anxiety of witnessing her suffering and feeling helpless? Was this the chilling, silent response of the physicians' shame? Which was experienced to the 14-year-old as her own shame.

We are all born needy, and it is arrogant and foolish to say otherwise. The question is not whether we have needs or not, but rather how we identify these needs and meet them. This is a tragic story of the innocence and the deep, deep hurt of a young girl who was invisible to her caregivers during a period of unimaginable, profound loss. There was no container for her emotional pain, and her humanity was not acknowledged. Her needs went underground and were still waiting to be heard when Susan came to see me ten years later. The physicians had observed her body and treated her in an objective, scientific way. They split the body from the soul in this young adolescent, and she felt it. They were able to cure her, but there was no healing.

The archetype of the orphan

Shame brings the intolerable experience of feeling orphaned or alone. As Susan grew older and chose the profession of healer herself, she still carried the physicians' shame from that experience. The resulting abandonment she felt in that moment with the physicians was triggered, retraumatizing Susan, as she re-experienced the loss of her mother and sister. Her need was to be seen, heard, and held in a safe emotional container.

The suffering of the physician is immense. The question I proposed earlier: Is there meaning in the suffering of the physician or is it meaningless? Dr. Ribi stated, "Suffering belongs to life" (Personal Communication, February 2018).

If this is so, which I believe it is, then there is a great need for the development of caring for the self of the physician. Not because physicians are different from any other human, but perhaps because their call may be greater in dealing with the life and death of human beings. The facade of the physician as being strong and untroubled is falling in a world that no longer has high regard for the most respected of all professions. We live in a time dominated by the lack of meaning, in which people have the capacity to connect more than ever reported in history, yet we also live in a time when relationships fall short as people experience a great need to belong to someone, some place, or thing more than ever before. This sense of belonging is difficult in a world that is hungry for power and money, which seems to have overtaken the realm of medical training and the art of medicine. It seems this is a world that suffers from spiritual depletion, emotional alienation, and personal isolation. Jung's words in his autobiography come to mind: "I am an orphan alone" (1963, 227). What do we do with our aloneness? Jungian analyst Janis Maxwell recently shared with me the following passage from Joseph Campbell (1991):

> The most powerful myths... display a balance between the severe and gentle aspects of the father, justice and mercy cooperating to the end that only the hero of the highest virtue shall become the vehicle of the highest energy. The story of Gethsemane and Calvary may be read as such a test and triumph; through His agony of going to the Father, the Only Son brought to the children of God the Fire of Redemption, so that on the day of Pentecost seven-times-seven days after the sublime reception by the Father of the Risen Son, the Spirit descended to man in Tongues of Flame.

References

Campbell, J. (1991). *The power of myth*. New York, NY: Anchor Publishing.

Fossum, M.A., & Mason, M.J. (1989). *Facing shame: Families in recovery*. New York, NY: W.W. Norton and Company.

Jung, C.G. (1963). *Memories, dreams, reflections*. Aniela Jaffé (Ed.). R. Winston & C. Winston (Trans.). New York, NY: Random House.

Chapter 12

Redeeming the voice of the physician through Jungian pathways

In middle of the journey of our days

I found that I was in a darksome wood—

The right road lost and vanished in the maze.

Dante Alighieri, The Divine Comedy

Although today's physician may be striving to carry the archetype of Asclepius, the current reality of Western medicine clouds this possibility, as the soul of medicine has been lost. Where might the physician find voice? Where is the world of medicine asleep, and how can it be awakened? This book has focused on the plight of physicians and how they have been anesthetized to the point of despair by a kingdom that has lost its way. Cut off from the homeland that they thought the world of medicine would offer, physicians have wandered, like Dante, into exile (Fox, 1988). The testaments they have shared with me reflect their sense of banishment from the realm that once honored their desire to be healers. Their stories reflect their deep sense of feeling homeless in their profession as well as hopeless and helpless in not knowing the way back to the kingdom of caring that called them initially. Thus, the archetype of the orphan has been constellated, which carries the sense of searching for the metaphorical king who can lead them. Unfortunately, their kingdom has been dying since the 1980s, when health care took a sudden turn toward economics at the expense of care and healing. In this shift, I believe the spark of the physician began to lose its light.

Where can redemption be found? I believe Jungian psychology holds the answer, for it has been my experience, through decades of listening to physicians' accounts, that their hunger has been sated through their exposure to a Jungian perspective in our work together.

The descent

Jung wrote of the search for purpose and meaning in life due to the loss of a religious attitude (Jung, 1966a). He suggested that cultivating a religious

DOI: 10.4324/9781003144502-12

attitude through contact with the numinous energy of the unconscious is a necessary component of the process of individuation. The process of working with the numinous energy of the unconscious has been transformative work, not only for me, but for the countless physicians with whom I have worked over the years, whom I have come to know as my analysands. I wish I could say it has been all joy. Parts of it have been joyful, but just as many parts have been as joyless as hard, dry, cracked earth when a gentle rain has been absent for too long. It has been a path of suffering for both the physicians and me, with loneliness as a constant companion—lonely for what, I am not always sure. There were times when I cried, cursed, and quit, only to begin again.

How is it that we begin again? The development of the totality of the personality and the shifting of control from the ego to the self is a terrifying journey, but it is the journey worth taking. How does one navigate these untraversed territories? Jung illuminated the image of the self that emerges from this process as imprinted with the imago Dei of which I wrote earlier in this text: "One can, then, explain the God-image... as a reflection of the self, or conversely, explain the self as imago Dei in man" (Jung, 1966a).

The pull toward alluring brilliance

The pursuit of the numinous, of the imago-Dei within, has been described in different ways: Hillman (1996) might call it the soul's code, or Campbell (2004) may find it suggesting, "Follow your bliss." Jesus called it "the way" (John 14:6 ESV), and Jung referred to it as the "true self" (1969, p. 37, para. 70). Whatever name one wants to use, this thread is the thing that holds one's life together and gives one a sense of meaning and purpose. We can never say that a life is worthless, but it is nonetheless true that the life that does not have this thing (whatever we call it) is an impoverished life. Today, as I pause, I can see a thread that has been woven that I have followed. I cannot say what another's thread is, nor do I know for sure what thread weaves through the life tapestry of any of the physicians whose stories I have shared, because none of us can do that for another person. Our own thread must be discovered by each of us. I believe that as we come to know that thread and hold dearly to it, all losses and sufferings (and there are many) will take on new and meaningful interpretations.

I am reminded of a concept presented by Christian theologian and philosopher Pseudo-Dionysius, the Areopagite, in the 6th century. He said we begin our spiritual journey thinking we are pulling on a chain that is attached to heaven. As we make our path through the years, we come to realize the chain we thought we were pulling is rather pulling us, toward its alluring brilliance (Pseudo-Dionysius, 1987). The thread that I have been holding has all along been holding me.

Active imagination to access the numinous

Active imagination is a process of working with the deep unconscious, using the capacity of the patient to go inside and experience their own deeper stories. I believe that what neurologists today call the "neuroplasticity of the brain" is what Jung was addressing when he introduced active imagination to the psychological world in the early 1900s. It is my hope that the modern-day frenzy of what is called the "new frontier of psychology" will be able to give due credit to the work of Jung, as he used this process in his own life and pioneered it in the therapeutic community as well. It is important to note, however, that Jung was not the originator of active imagination. He attributed the beginnings of such activities to primitive humans who depended on their imaginations for their very survival in dealing with the numinous. Active imagination produces a coherent series of images of which the dream may only reveal fragments. Jung encouraged analysts and their patients to move with caution toward this depth of encounter with the unconscious, adding that analysts should only accompany analysands if they are determined to go where no other path will fulfill their need (Jung, 1969).

In my work with physicians, active imagination is a highly effective tool, as it helps move the physician from the intellect to the imagination, allowing the possibility of an opening to the numinous through spontaneous images. In fact, Jung wrote,

> The main interest of my work is not connected with the treatment of neuroses but rather with the approach to the numinous. But the fact is that the approach to the numinous is the real therapy and inasmuch as you attain to the numinous experiences, you are released from the curse of pathology. (Jung, 1973, pp. 376–377)

In my personal process, I was led to the numinous by the dream image of the snakes in a personal confrontation of two white cobras facing me eye to eye. I explored what the unconscious might be asking more fully through an active imagination exercise. By trusting the process of spontaneous discovery, I was able to realize the symbolism of the snake entering my body as an instinctual form and exiting my body in a spiritual form as the holy dove feathers forming a complete circle. I wondered how the snake may be related to my soul and found myself more open to the possibility that my path would involve healing. Jungian analyst Jeffrey Raff (2006) suggested,

> Imagination brings higher meaning of the spirit into the soul and raises lower concrete reality to the soul through the creation of images. It is a supreme way of knowing reality and completely free... imagination is real and brings into union the three dimensions of reality: soul, body and spirit.

The body is where one can discover the newfound energy of the animus or anima. In this process, one must develop a container strong enough for the new creativity that brings forth healing. For the physician, healing is often experienced through guided imagery, taking them back to their childhood to contact the child archetype. Shortly thereafter, the physician is able to participate in active imagination allowing them the opportunity to experience the numinous.

This imaginal ability seems to have been a gift of mine from childhood that has continued throughout my life, allowing me to see new possibilities in waking life, leading to the unification of body, soul, and spirit, snakes and doves, and anima and animus. For physicians, the call to imagination seems to be for uniting eros and logos in the service of creating a new medical model. For Jung, a creative, active imagination is an autonomous process that holds the possibility of accessing the unconscious. For me, creativity and imagination are inherent in my deep connection to nature, which seems to have a consciousness of its own.

Nature as the great mother

The deepest experiences of my early experience in life were tied to nature itself, as I was fortunate to live close to the land. Generations of ranchers, horses, and cattle are in my bones. I grew up listening to the first sounds of spring coming from the geese as they flew from south to the north. I learned about the crocus and daffodils blooming while snow lay on the ground and knew spring would soon be arriving. I knew when the ground was ready to be tilled, the color of wheat when it was ripe for harvest, and that the first glistening of frost meant winter was on its way. By the age of six, I understood that when a seed was planted in the cold dark earth waiting in the fertile darkness for life to be born, in the meantime, it needed water, the warmth of the sun, and fertilizer. I understood that earth was to be honored, respected, listened to.

Nature became my refuge from disappointment or hurt. I came to view nature as the greatest artist who greeted me with the softness of a gentle spring breeze or comfort at the base of a giant oak tree against which I would lean, imagining how deeply its roots might be, while looking to see how far its mighty limbs reached into the sky. This was my first experience of Beauty. Today, I would say this was my first experience of God through nature's art. The clear blue sky and the vastness of Texas ranchland seemed to hold it all. The sounds of the rain on the tin roof of a barn, the cry of a newborn calf in the morning, and the sound of my horse's hooves filled my soul, connecting me to something larger than myself, which one can only know by experience. For me this was Beauty. This was Nature. The first image of the Holy given to us.

I knew little of art by pencil or paintbrush. In my world, clay was to be molded from the mud in between my toes as I sat on the riverbank listening to the calming sound of flowing water. As a child, I delighted in creating images of wild horses, princesses, and kingdoms in the clouds as they floated overhead. Perhaps I was participating in my first active imagination long before I knew of such a thing. It was here that I would unknowingly experience an important tool in the craft of soul making, even before I knew its name: Imagination. Jung often referenced the value of the imagination and play of a child, which he practiced in his many days at Bollingen. It was as a child that I first imagined being a physician. It was also in the world of play that I was wounded as I "played doctor" with my classmate. It was imagination that led me to the tree when I was diagnosed with adenocarcinoma, where I meekly claimed, "The same DNA that is in you, is in me." For me, nature is the divine life force.

When I speak of nature or the natural life force of me as a woman, I am reminded of what Clarissa Pinkola Estes describes as a Wild Woman:

> Within every woman there is a wild and natural creature, a powerful force, filled with good instincts, passionate creativity, and ageless knowing. Her name is Wild Woman, but she is an endangered species. Though the gifts of the wildest nature come to us at birth, society's attempt to "civilize "us into rigid roles has plundered this treasure, and muffled the deep, life giving messages of our own souls. Without Wild Woman we become over-domesticated, fearful, uncreative, trapped. (Estes, 1992, p. xxx)

Multiple paths to the numinous

In my experience with physicians and others, not everyone can participate in active imagination or live so close to the land. There are still multiple avenues to accessing the numinous: Art, poetry, relatedness, science, dancing, any expression of the self in an art form. For Jung, participating in this life force experience required holding onto the essence of his childhood self and experience into adulthood with a trust of the reality of the interior self—a task that he said few could manage. He added,

> Here I am alluding to a problem that is far more significant that these few simple words would seem to suggest: mankind is, in essentials, psychologically still in a state of childhood—a stage that cannot be skipped. The vast majority needs authority, guidance, law. This fact cannot be overlooked. The Pauline overcoming of the law falls only to the man who knows how to put his soul in the place of conscience. Very few are capable of this. And these few tread this path from inner

necessity, not to say suffering, for it is sharp as the edge of a razor. (Jung, 1966a, p. 239, para. 401)

Today, I can look back and see that I seemed to have been called to engage the archetype of the orphan and to dwell in the presence of kings whom I would come to know as physicians. I would listen to them as they taught me about their calling, courage, perseverance, and human life and dignity. I watched their kingdom grow, only to bear witness to its ongoing demise. I recognize a hallelujah here, for in the death of the old is the invitation for the new to come. It is clear to me that from a Jungian perspective, accessing the unconscious involves many modalities: Active imagination, relating, writing, music, dreams, fairy tales, creating art, and acknowledging the conscious-ness of nature, among others. I have witnessed the power of using these tools in the physician's lives with whom I have been privileged to work

The healer's journey

As I contemplated the contents of this chapter, I remembered my beginning—my early traumas and the call that began on the day of my birth as a black baby. My recurrent childhood dream was of *me being in a mesquite tree with rattlesnakes at the bottom trying to come up the tree.* At 19, I had another dream: *All was black with just one star coming toward me.* When I shared this dream with my mother, she said, "This is an important dream." Curiously, as I wrote this paragraph in an active imagination one morning, a spark came out of the darkness—the same image as that in my dream, almost 50 years ago.

I questioned, *what does this darkness mean and where is the spark?* The symbols in my dream that I longed to understand were perhaps leading me to a destiny that involved healing. Dreams embody psyche's urge toward newness—new stories, new myths. Contextual amplifications and associa-tions bring to the dream images of what has been. Perhaps, relative to this book, my dream presages the falling of the kingdom of medicine and points to what is coming; perhaps the dream maker was asking me to be a parti-cipant or co-creator with these physicians in the next chapter of my life. Then, in the darkness of a night of deep sleep, a dream of one of those tiny sparks made itself known with all the uncomfortableness of childbirth. Was I now being asked to be the mother of the spark? Is that what Jung meant when he said we become the mother of God?

I wondered, could I really trust Jung and his teachings, which suggest that "in reality, the work of art grows out of the artist as a child... and arises from the unconscious depths?" (1966a, p. 103, para. 159). Could I stand with the physician as we moved away from the collective, separating from the herd? Could I continue to hold space for the physician entering into this creative process? According to Jung, when one is asked to do so, the ar-chetype of the hero figure is making its presence known as "a quasi-human being who symbolizes the ideas, forms, and forces which grip and mold the soul" (1967, p. 178, para. 259). How would we journey from the psychological movement of the old expression of consciousness to a new one of greater meaning? Who and what would help birth this process between the ego and the archetypal Self, not only for me, but for my traveling companions as well, the physicians and their patients?

Where the spirit enters

I am still working with that dream to discover its meaning, moving me from the two little black snakes on the east side of a pond to the two large vertical iridescent snakes on the west side of the pond, keeping in mind Jung's proposition that a dream can mean anything. The calling of the confrontation of my soul was at hand. How does one take the *prima materia* and begin? How does one become a good Jungian analyst or a good physician? What do these two have in common? From a purely psychological/archetypal point of view, Guggenbühl-Craig (2015) identified three archetypes that answer the question adequately. The first archetype is that of the healer, the second is the reality, the work of art grows out of the artist as a child... and arises from the unconscious depths" (1966a). And the third is the alchemist. For the sake of this book, I have substituted wounded healer for shaman, suggesting that the woundedness is the place of the call. Rumi (1995) wrote that the "wound" is the place "where the light enters you."

In the Native American tradition, the old Navajo grandmother says that into every Navajo rug is woven a purposeful flaw in the beautiful tapestry, as the Navajo also believe the flaw is where the spirit enters. It seems we are facing the flaw in healthcare searching for the spirit that might replace the value of money with the value of human relationships.

Entering the shadowlands

Initially, I did not want to pursue my dream. I was afraid of it, yet I could not let it go. As in the tale of Jonah and the whale, I felt I must go to Nineveh (Jonah 1–4, NIV). I feared that to refuse to do so would perhaps bring a depression or dark night of the soul. I had been given a story that needed to be told. Though I much preferred to keep my story to myself, quietly working with the physicians in the sacred container or temenos of my office, I feared that, from a Jungian perspective, my ego's need for security might lead to certain death of my inner life. I did not understand that even the surrender to the call would be its own hell, as I was afraid to enter into the depths of the unconscious world. In the end, the unconscious world of symbols and images with no linear path to follow became simply a journey to be made. I was often reminded by Dr. Ribi to "face the image—stay with the image" (Personal Communication, February 2018). He would then ask what I would do with an image in real life? I always responded that I would "Run, Dr. Ribi, I would run!" but wherever I would go, there I was. I was running from me, but I could not get away from me, whatever me was. Indeed, this is a familiar path for the intuitive, but I now know I was being asked to stay with the image, face it, interact with it, just as I was asking the physicians to find their symbols as they came to understand the archetype of the healer—more specifically, the wounded healer. The physicians also had to face the transformative work of the psyche. Their stagnation would be challenged by the creative process, which would ask them to emerge into a new form: The physician as healer.

I decided to face the snakes—a conscious decision, a decision that would change the course of my life. This decision was to face my body, sexuality, and eros, as denoted by the two black snakes, as well as spirituality and logos, as shown by the two iridescent snakes. This meant a descent into the shadow. Jung provided a path to examine the individuation process in his essay "The Relations Between the Ego and the Unconscious" (1966b), in which he states that those aspects of self that have been repressed or ignored by the ego will emerge in the form of the shadow. It is difficult for all of us to integrate our shadow content, but perhaps more so for the physician who often has identified with God-like projections from the patient. Jung emphatically stated that the only honest and effective way of dealing with the shadow is to admit the shadow into the encounter consciously. In my own historical roots of Native American Spirituality, a basic tenet is "The greater the sun, the greater the shadow."

Shadow is difficult for the physician and for me because of the very connotation of the words *darkness* and *unknown*. We had to understand that darkness can hold both negative and positive aspects. In fact, the alchemist would tell us that these are the base materials needed to begin the process of refining the *prima materia* into gold by the aid of fire. Yes, it was the shadowlands that needed the most attention for both the physicians and me. Often the shadow is encountered in dreams as a person of the same gender as the dreamer but with opposite characteristics. However, the snake symbols in my dream connected me not only to the healing spirit guides of Native American Culture but also to the medical culture as represented by the caduceus worn by the physician, which symbolizes the healing and the transformation of the body. It was, in fact, the symbol of the snake that I no longer could ignore.

As I began to lean into what this might mean for me, I was reminded of David Whyte's poem "Sweet Darkness":

When your eyes are tired,
the world is tired also.
When your vision has gone,
no part of the world can find you.
Time to go into the dark

where the night has eyes
to recognize its own.
There you can be sure
you are not beyond love.
The dark will be your home
tonight.
The night will give you a horizon
further than you can see.
You must learn one thing.
The world was made to be free in.
Give up all the other worlds
except the one to which you belong.
Sometimes it takes darkness and the sweet
confinement of your aloneness
to learn
anything or anyone
that does not bring you alive
is too small for you.

References

Alighieri, D. (1884). *The divine comedy of Dante Alighieri, the inferno/* James Roman Sibbald (Trans.). Edinburgh, Scotland: David Douglas, 1884. Ebook # 41537. https://www.gutenberg.org/files/41537/41537-h/41537-h.htm

Campbell, J. (2004). *Pathways to bliss: Mythology and personal transformation.* In D. Kudler (Ed.). Novato, CA: New World Library.

Estes, C.P. (1992). *Women who Run with the Wolves: Myths and stories of the wild woman archetype.* New York, NY: Ballantine Books.

Fox, M. (1988). *The coming of the cosmic Christ.* San Francisco, CA: Harper San Francisco.

Guggenbühl-Craig, A. (2015). *Power in the helping professions.* M. Gubitz (Trans.). Dallas, TX: Spring.

Hillman, J. (1996). *The soul's code: In search of character and calling.* New York, NY: Ballantine Books.

Jung, C. G. (1966a). Psychology and literature. In H. Read, M. Fordham, G. Adler, & W. McGuire (Eds.), *The collected works of C. G. Jung: Vol. 15. The spirit in man, art, and literature.* R.F.C. Hull (Trans.). Princeton, NJ: Princeton University Press.

Jung, C.G. (1966b). The relations between the ego and the unconscious. In H. Read, M. Fordham, G. Adler, & W. McGuire (Eds.), *The collected works of C. G. Jung: Vol. 7. Two essays in analytical psychology.* R.F.C. Hull (Trans.). Princeton, NJ: Princeton University Press.

Jung, C.G. (1967). *The collected works of C. G. Jung: Vol.5. Symbols of transformation.* H. Read, M. Fordham, G. Adler, & W. McGuire (Eds.). R.F.C. Hull (Trans.). Princeton, NJ: Princeton University Press.

Jung, C.G. (1968). *The collected works of C. G. Jung: Vol. 9ii. Aion.* H. Read, M. Fordham, G. Adler, & W. McGuire (Eds.). R.F.C. Hull (Trans.). Princeton, NJ: Princeton University Press.

Jung, C.G. (1969). The transcendent function. In H. Read, M. Fordham, G. Adler, & W. McGuire (Eds.), *The collected works of C. G. Jung: Vol. 8. The structure and dynamics of the psyche.* R.F.C. Hull (Trans.). Princeton, NJ: Princeton University Press.

Jung, C.G. (1973). *Letters, vol. 1: 1906–1950.* G. Adler, A. Jaffé, & R.F.C. Hull (Trans.). Princeton, NJ: Princeton University Press.

Pseudo-Dionysius. (1987). The divine names. In *Pseudo-Dionysius: The complete works.* C. Luibheid & P. Rorem (Trans.). New York, NY: Paulist Press.

Raff, J. (2006). *The practice of ally work: Meeting and partnering with your spirit guide in the imaginal world.* Berwick, ME: Nicholas-Hayes.

Rumi, J. ā.-d. (1995). *The essential Rumi.* C. Barks (Trans.). San Francisco, CA: Harper San Francisco.

Whyte, D. (1977). *The house of belonging.* Langley, WA: Many Rivers Press.

Chapter 13

The offering

The gift you carry for others is not an attempt to save the world but to fully belong to it. It's not possible to save the world by trying to save it. You need to find what is genuinely yours to offer the world before you can make it a better place. Discovering the unique gift to bring to your community is your greatest opportunity and challenge. The offering of that gift... your true self... is the most you can do to love and serve the world... and it is all the world needs.

Bill Plokin (2003) Soulcraft: Crossing into the Mysteries of
Nature and Psyche

Jung's innate propensity to live a symbolic life became an important aspect of analytical psychology that has informed my own process as well as my work with physicians. I have come to realize that the issue of the ego consciously committing to the symbolic life is not a scientific question. I have been asking physicians to explore another side of the psyche having more in common with religious and artistic traditions than with science. In Jung's *Memories, Dreams, Reflections*, a crucial passage stands out for me:

I took great care to try to understand every single image, every item of my psychic inventory, and to classify them scientifically—so far as this was possible—and above all, to realize them in actual life. That is what we usually neglect to do. We allow the images to rise up, and maybe we wonder about them, but that is all. We do not take the trouble to understand them, let alone draw ethical conclusions from them. This stopping short conjures up the negative effects of the unconscious. It is equally a grave mistake to think that it is enough to gain some understanding of the images and that knowledge can here make a halt. Insight into them must be converted into an ethical obligation. Not to do so is to fall prey to the power principle, and this produces dangerous effects which are destructive not only to others but even to the knower. The images of the unconscious place a great responsibility upon a man. Failure to understand them or a shirking of

DOI: 10.4324/9781003144502-13

ethical responsibility, deprives him of his wholeness and imposes a painful
fragmentariness on his life. (Jung, 1963, 192)

A commitment to the image, or the symbolic life, is the work of the ongoing
process of individuation. The undeveloped components of my personality
structure that had been sent away were asking to be known, to be integrated,
in order to continue the individuation process. What form was this integration of the shadow going to take in my conscious life? Along with my
shadow was the shadow of the physician who routinely presented in my
office, asking to be known, asking to be integrated. The reclamation of the
call of healing involves the wholeness of the healer: His logic and his eros,
science, and soul. They are not separate, and the attempts to split off eros in
the physician reflect the tragic one-sidedness of medicine today.

The wholeness of the healer is found not only in the reclamation of the
feeling function, but the redemption of his suffering and shame. Leonard
Cohen's song "Hallelujah" (1985) presents this idea with these poignant lyrics:

> Now I've heard there was a secret chord,
> That David played and it pleased the Lord,
> But you don't really care for music, do you?
> It goes like this, the fourth, the fifth
> The minor fall, the major lift
> The baffled king, composing Hallelujah.

As well as

> There's a blaze of light in every word
> It doesn't matter which you heard
> The holy or the broken hallelujah.

Most of my life, I have simply wanted to live in the "hallelujah," discarding
the brokenness or, worse yet, claiming that I was broken. I felt shame, true
to the shadow of the American collective that needed to stay hidden, for
ours is a culture that values victory, perfection, and light. The last line above
in Cohen's song holds the opposites that I was being asked to live
throughout my life. I realized that these opposites of holy and brokenness
were actually one. There is a sacredness in brokenness. Perhaps this is the
secret chord of David referenced by Cohen. This lyric suggests that both
aspects of the hallelujah are parts of a whole that have equal value to one
another. Could the rigid, scientific environment of medical schools be open
to hearing the secret chord to which so many physicians I have worked with
have been so responsive?

Notably, physicians are asked to live in the perfection of the "hallelujah" with no way to deal with their own brokenness. The crux of Cohen's message is that being vulnerable is uncomfortable, whether one is celebrated or in despair and we must embrace both, maintaining the tension of the opposites so that something new may emerge.

References

Cohen, L. (1985). *Hallelujah. On various positions [CD]*. USA: Columbia.

Jung, C.G. (1963). *Memories, dreams, reflections*. Aniela Jaffé (Ed.). R. Winston & C. Winston (Trans.). New York, NY: Random House.

Plokin, B. (2003). *Soulcraft: Crossing into the mysteries of nature and psyche*. Novato, CA: New World Library.

Epilogue

As I draw close to the end of this book, it is with gratitude that I sit today and look at the black baby doll that hangs in the center of my office. Why did I keep her all those many years ago hidden away? How did she survive the fire?

My memory takes me to 1986, when I was attending my first group therapy session listening to the ideas of Jung. When I initially sat down, the group's facilitator asked me why I had come. I replied, "I want to become a woman of grace." It was fortunate that I did not know what was involved in the development of grace, or I might have run away. He just smiled and welcomed me. It was then that I was introduced to the child within. The psychologist's way of working with the group opened a new world to me, for which I will forever be grateful. I sat in that therapy group for one year without saying a word. I just listened. As I listened, I drew images as they came from the unconscious.

I look at the picture shown in Figure 14.1, and I see the rising of the feminine. I drew seven trees, all evergreens, with roots that became the hair of the tribal primal-looking woman under the trees with the black woman, perhaps the Black Madonna with raised hands at the bottom of the page. Today, I know this was the beginning of the emergence of the divine feminine in my life, which was a concept unknown to me at that time. I studied this picture, and as I looked at the black baby doll and then at the painting of the Black Madonna, for the first time, I wondered: Was this the gift my father gave me in the form of the black baby, the Black Madonna of whom he was certainly not aware? Was the struggle with patriarchal parents necessary for me to experience life as I was asked to live it? Was I being called to be a healer of the dark and broken places of life? Was the spark there all along as my black baby was thrown away, only to be found in the rubbish and debris of transformative fire? Was it that fire, the "creative fire," that traveled up my spine?

This was not the first time that I had experienced this deep awareness of Sophia's presence. Often, it occurs when the sudden recognition of her radiant presence is felt—when I experience nature and feel something that

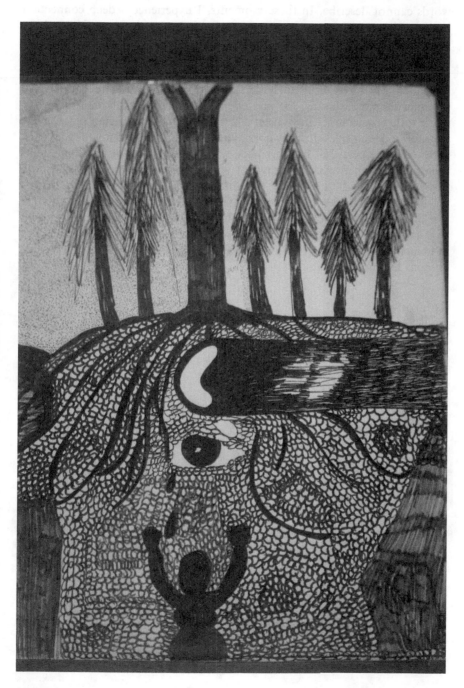

Figure 14.1 The rising of the feminine.

words cannot describe. In these moments, I experience a deep connection between the vast beauty of the universe and the goodness of Divine Life. When I discovered that the Greek word for *wisdom* is *Sophia*, she took on a very personal and intimate connection with me. She had been there all along—a black baby, a medicine bag, a horse, Ishmael, the Black Madonna, and Sophia. I have come to understand my calling and life path as the groundwork preparing me for the redemption of what truly matters in my work with physicians. I have been a witness to how a Jungian process has transformed their lives. It is my hope that the next thread in my life's journey will weave a tapestry of healing made whole as the weft of the divine feminine interlocks between the strands of Western medicine, thereby redeeming physicians through the divine feminine. I am most inspired by Jung's teaching that a healer may take comfort in the fact that "He is not just working for this particular patient... but for himself as well and his own soul, and in so doing he is perhaps laying an infinitesimal grain in the scales of humanity's soul. Small and indivisible as this contribution may be, it is yet an opus magnum..." (Jung, 1954).

Reference

Jung, C.G. (1954). *The collected works of C.G. Jung: Vol. 16. The practice of psychotherapy.* H. Read, M. Fordham, G. Adler, & W. McGuire (Eds.). R.F.C. Hull (Trans.). Princeton, NJ: Princeton University Press.

Index

Printed in the United States
by Baker & Taylor Publisher Services

Printed in the United States
by Baker & Taylor Publisher Services